Inte[...]

Fasting for Women

The Complete Guide to Healthy Eating for Weight Loss and Body Cleansing

Author: Joleen Donovan

Table of Contents

Book Description:

Are you curious about the lifestyle benefits of intermittent fasting? For the modern, on-the-go woman, few other eating practices have proven to be so good for your health and wellbeing.

It's not a diet. It's not a fad. There's real science behind intermittent fasting. Best of all, it suits the fast-paced lifestyle you lead. If you struggle with weight, nutrition, blood sugar regulation and stress – intermittent fasting could be the discovery that helps you change your life for the better.

In *Intermittent Fasting for Women,* I walk you through what it is, how it works and more importantly why it's one of the most promising lifestyle changes you can adopt in 2019. If you want to look healthier, thinner and younger than you have in years – the secret is inside this guide!

In this book you'll discover:

- The long, important history of intermittent fasting

- The proven science behind why it works and why it's critical for human health

- What exactly changes in your body and mind, when you start intermittent fasting

- The 7 most powerful intermittent fasting methods

- What you can eat, and what you should never, ever eat

- How to get started and problems you might have to overcome

If you're tired of your eating habits and need a drastic positive change, this is the best idea you've ever had. The lessons in this book will benefit every part of your life.

Start your intermittent fasting journey and adopt a lifestyle that is making women stronger, happier and healthier than they have ever been. It begins with this guide, and a plan.

Discover how to fast intermittently with this step-by-step guide.

Buy it now, the secrets are inside!

Introduction

Many people think that the term "intermittent fasting" refers to a diet, but this is not a diet. Instead, it is rather an eating habit that people adopt that gives them guidance on when they should eat – this allows the digestive system to take a break from processing and digesting food continuously.

For many people, this type of dietary habit seems unhealthy. There are a lot of people who are scared of adopting this pattern of eating because they think that they would starve themselves. This, however, is a common myth that has been told about intermittent fasting.

This particular dietary-scheduling technique has been used since ancient times. Numerous studies have been carried out to determine how the technique interacts with the human body, and several advantages have already been noted.

An important fact that you should know when it comes to discussing this method of eating is that, since it is not classified as a diet, it will not decide the types of food that you will be eating. It is your role to decide what you want to eat. A healthy, balanced diet that is filled with foods high in essential nutrients will, of course, result in more benefits compared to stuffing yourself with hamburgers and pizza as soon as the clock strikes five, or whatever time your eating cycle starts. When opting for fast foods and other food options that are very high in carbohydrates, weight loss may not be a particular benefit that you experience when following this diet.

Planning exercise days well is important. If you practice high-intensity workouts on the fasting day, you will feel exhausted, and your muscles will be under a lot of stress, which is not good when you are trying to shape and enhance. Also, to get those well-established and toned muscles, drink plenty of water (at least eight glasses, but this is the minimum amount we need) and remember to combine protein, carbohydrates, and fat before and after training to help your muscles grow. Take the recommendations for gradual entry into the process of fasting and become one step closer to changing your whole life and becoming happier and satisfied with your visual appearance and health.

Thanks for downloading this book. It's my firm belief that it will provide you with all the answers to your questions.

Chapter 1
What Is Intermittent Fasting?

What Is Intermittent Fasting?

The word intermittent means irregular, broken, or discontinuous and the term fasting refers to going without food for some time. Therefore, intermittent fasting entails cycling between periods of eating and fasting.

Intermittent fasting is not a 'diet' in the conventional sense in that it does not tell you what to eat. However, it does tell you when to eat and when to fast. This is why intermittent fasting is often referred to as a pattern of eating. As a pattern of eating, it has:

An Eating Window

The eating window is the time in which you are supposed to eat. For example, if you have an 8-hour eating window, this means that you can only eat something within those eight hours. As such, you can decide to eat two meals or three meals or even eat snacks in between the meals. If you don't exceed the eating time, you will still be within the eating window. However, once the eating window elapses, you need to stop eating and enter the fasting period.

The Fasting Period

The fasting period refers to the duration of time you will stay without consuming any calories. This time can be anywhere between 16-36 hours. The good news is that you can arrange the fasting period to encompass the eight or more hours you will be asleep. This way, it will feel like you are 'fasting' for a shorter period. Still, if you are having trouble going through the fasting period, you can have some zero-calorie beverages such as:

Tea - Tea, especially green tea, is something you will want to keep around. Apart from reducing hunger pangs, tea helps reduce LDL cholesterol and that stubborn abdominal fat. However, you must drink it as it is. Don't add any sweeteners that contain calories.

Coffee - Coffee is another beverage you can indulge in during your fasting period. It is calorie-free, and it comes with a healthy dose of antioxidants. What's more, coffee is said to boost your metabolism. As such, it is good for weight loss. However, you need to monitor your intake as some people experience things such as an upset stomach or a racing heart when they drink coffee.

Water–Water is one of those beverages that you must drink whether you are fasting or not. Nevertheless, it would be prudent to increase your intake during intermittent fasting. This is because fasting detoxifies your body. These toxins need to be flushed out, and water helps your body remove them. Also, water rejuvenates you and makes you feel full, which in turn helps you go through your day without feeling drained.

Apart from drinking various zero-calorie beverages, you can also pass the time by chewing gum. Most gums happen to be made with sugar alcohols, and they contain no calories. They can come in handy especially when you want to give your mouth something to do. When you chew gum, you keep hunger at bay by tricking your brain into thinking you are chewing, hence eating.

Chapter 2
Intermittent Fasting History

What makes intermittent fasting different than any other forms of dieting is that it is not a modern fad; rather it is an age-old technique that has been rediscovered and brought back into the limelight by certain people. It is like Yoga of the world of food.

You will be surprised to learn that people have been fasting since ancient days, perhaps right from the beginning of the human race. If human bodies and evolution are to be considered, eating many meals and snacks throughout the day is neither necessary for survival, nor are they good for health. In fact, an excess of food, like the excess of anything can be extremely harmful to the body. In ancient times, the availability of food was unpredictable and irregular. It was difficult to gather and store food. Seasonal changes too made it difficult to come across food often. For instance, it was easy to get food in summers; however, it became excessively scarce in winters. This phenomenon of fluctuating food and food sources continued until the modern era for everyone except the upper class. In the last century, droughts, famines, wars, diseases, disorders, etc. led to the depletion of food sources. All of these led to starvation and sometimes death as well. It is no wonder that one of those famines is one of the Four Ushers of Apocalypse.

The history of fasting can be roughly divided into three eras - ancient, medieval, and modern. Let us have a look at all three one by one.

Ancient History

The age of scrounging and gathering ended when humans discovered agriculture, perhaps by accident or observation. Once we discovered and developed agriculture, the incidents of famine went down. Agriculture led to the development of societies and culture and religion soon followed. Soon, people all over the world realized that going hungry for a limited period was beneficial for the health of your mind and body. This was then the first instance of periodic fasting. Periodic fasting became a staple of almost all the religions in the world. Forced starvation was replaced by controlled and voluntary fasting as it made people calm, happy, and healthy. It is no wonder that fasting was often called 'detox' 'purification' 'purge' 'ritualistic cleaning' in ancient times. The ancients believed that fasting held the power to clean the body and the soul and that it could help them to please God(s).

Spiritual Fasting

Religious or spiritual fasting still enjoys a strong position in all major religions. Buddha, Christ, and Prophet Mohammad all believed in the power of fasting and advised their followers to fast periodically. It should be noted that fasting as a practice developed intrinsically and independently in varied cultures and religions. This means that people all over realized that fasting had some benefits. Christians follow with Lent; Hindus with various fasts and the Muslims followed Ramadan fasts. Similarly, the Buddhists and Jain came up with certain eating times that they must follow. All of these are types of fasting.

Fasting for Health in the Ancient Times

If we are to consider the history of fasting for health benefits, we should be grateful to Ayurveda and the ancient Greeks. Ayurveda, I.e., the ancient medical science from India called for various forms of fasts and foods for different ailments and general wellbeing. Hippocrates aka the father of Modern Medicine also wrote a lot about fasting and obesity. Obesity was on the rise in the times of Hippocrates in ancient Greece. This was due to the lavish lifestyle and lack of health routines for the royalty. Hippocrates observed the correlation between obesity and early deaths and advised exercise and diet for obese people. The diet he advised included healthy food items and most prominently eating once a day only. After Hippocrates, Plutarch, the great historian, too understood the importance of fasting. Great thinkers such as Plato and Aristotle followed this.

The ancient Greeks believed fasting could improve mental and cognitive abilities and thought it could help them solve problems and puzzles with ease. While this sounds a bit preposterous, try to imagine how bloated and uncomfortable you feel after having a large meal. Meals make you lethargic as your body focuses its energy on the digestive system. You feel excessively sleepy and often doze off after a heavy meal. Some people call this condition a sleep coma. In contrast, if you avoid eating food for some time, you feel far sharper, active, and attuned to the atmosphere. Mind you, this is no accident; it's an evolutionary effect. In the Stone Age, our senses became sharper when food was scarce.

Medieval Times

Even in medieval times, the popularity of fasting did not wane; rather it continued to grow. Paracelsus, a Swiss-German physician who is well known as the father of toxicology, was a proponent of intermittent fasting. He was a firm believer of the theory that anything in excess can prove to be lethal and advised fasting for wellness. One of the founding fathers of the USA, Benjamin Franklin was a proponent of intermittent fasting. A man of many talents, Franklin was a polymath who was well-versed with many arts and sciences. Famous author Mark Twain too was a supporter of fasting for health.

Modern History of Fasting

While the rise of intermittent fasting as a regular diet is a recent phenomenon, fasting, in general, continued its journey from medieval times to modern times. References to fasting can be found as early as the late 1800s. Interestingly fasting developed as a form of entertainment in the late 1800s and early 1900s. The fad died though, thankfully.

Fasting became a staple of medical literature around the early 1900s. Journal of Biological Chemistry defined fasting as a safe and effective way of losing weight and reducing obesity. However, obesity was perhaps the last thing on the minds of people in the early 20th century. The world was changing rapidly, and wars and famines had become commonplace. People were dying for epidemics and starvation all over. With the rise of obesity in the 21st century, fasting once again became popular.

Fasting and Evolution

Fasting was a part of human evolution, and our body and mind are used and perhaps require regular periods of fasts. As most of the citizens of the developed and developing nations have access to ample food regularly, we have almost forgotten about fasting, and it is no wonder that some people look down upon it. Still, intermittent fasting is becoming popular as more and more people see positive results.

Chapter 3
Science Behind Intermittent Fasting

While every diet and fitness addition into your life comes with upsides and downsides, intermittent fasting has more pros than cons. If you approach intermittent fasting with an open mind, you'll find that it can help you reach your weight loss goals. In the next part more will be shared about the science behind intermittent fasting and what you can do about your hunger while fasting.

There is plenty of information and research that backs up intermittent fasting. As fasting is not a new thing, extensive research can be found on this topic. Intermittent fasting may soon become a fad, but thankfully it is a fad that is based on science. While much of the research on fasting has been done on animals, the science is still promising.

Fasting is not a new phenomenon. Fasting has been shown in the past to help the body to reset and clear the mind. Interestingly, science goes far beyond that. While there are several different theories as to why intermittent fasting works, one fascinating theory that has been well-researched is that intermittent fasting puts your body's cells under mild stress. When these cells are stressed, they keep adapting and can fight off disease better. Stress is something that often carries a negative connotation.

On the contrary, stress is not inherently a bad thing. When you put your body under stress, positive results can occur. Think of when you exercise hard. You are exhausted and tired, but once your muscles recover, they are stronger. Research has shown that your body's cells respond to intermittent fasting very similar to exercise.

The reason you will lose weight while intermittent fasting can be attributed to a few different causes. For one, it will be much easier to eat fewer calories in the limited eating window. If you are eating on alternate days, during a window period, or skipping certain meals, you will tend to be consuming fewer calories than when you were eating multiple meals throughout the day. Another reason you may lose weight while fasting is because when you stop eating for an extended period, your body goes into its adipose tissue fat cells for energy. Ketones are released into the bloodstream that carries fat, and you end up losing your body fat through your urine. Research also shows that short-term fasting increases your metabolism speed. Your metabolism is what digests your food. When it works faster, it burns more calories, leading to more weight loss. While many other diets may limit your calorie intake, intermittent fasting does both things. You increase the calories you expend (by boosting your metabolism), and you also decrease the calories you eat. This creates a large calorie deficit. If you exercise on top of intermittent fasting, your calorie deficit becomes larger, and you will lose even more weight.

Intermittent fasting did not become a craze just because of weight loss. Intermittent fasting is popular amongst many already fit individuals because of the other benefits it comes with. One of these benefits is reducing the chance of insulin resistance. Type two diabetes is on the rise. Research says that intermittent fasting leads to a drop in blood sugar levels. Fasting, insulin was seen to drop as much as 20-30% and fasting blood sugar dropped by 3-6%. When you have lower insulin and blood sugar levels, you are at a lower risk for developing insulin resistance, which leads to type two diabetes.

If you are looking for anti-aging benefits, intermittent fasting may be the diet for you, too. Our bodies go through a process called oxidative stress. Oxidative stress leads to aging and many of the chronic diseases that we see on the rise today. Harmful free radicals react with our body's proteins and DNA and damage them which leads to these diseases and aging. However, studies have shown that intermittent fasting increases our body's ability to attack these harmful free radicals. This can help us to combat the effects of aging.

Fasting is also good for the heart. It's no surprise that cardiovascular disease is currently the number one killer in many countries. Intermittent fasting can help stabilize the brain's hormones and brings about better heart health. Fasting can reduce the risk of heart problems with risk factors such as LDL cholesterol, blood triglycerides, blood sugar levels, and inflammation levels lowered. If you have high cholesterol or are on medication for cholesterol and high blood pressure, intermittent fasting could lead to you dropping this medication.

While not proven in humans yet, intermittent fasting has shown impressive benefits in preventing cancer in animal studies. When these animals underwent intermittent fasting, they survived longer and had a reduction in symptoms from their tumors. Cancer is a disease that is not entirely understood and any research showing that this diet can help prevent it should be taken seriously. There was also a study that looked at humans going through chemotherapy. They found that the individuals who followed an intermittent fasting diet had fewer side effects from the chemotherapy. More research will need to be studied to understand fasting's relationship with cancer, but so far it seems to be very positive.

There have many good effects shown throughout research on intermittent fasting but how does it work? How does intermittent fasting cause all these great benefits?

Just as calories from vegetables are better than calories from chocolate cake, the timing of meal consumption can affect how a human body stores it most efficiently. Usually, when we eat something, our metabolism spends hours burning through this food and digesting it. As the stomach digests this food, it will either use the energy or store the energy as fat. Hence, for someone constantly eating throughout the day, the body is going to use the nearest energy source. It is going to burn the calories of what was just eaten instead of the stored energy from body fat. It doesn't need body fat because it is constantly getting a new stream of energy from the food that is being consumed 3 or more times a day. With intermittent fasting, the body is not provided with consistent food at every few hour intervals. Hence, with the body realizing it is not receiving any food, it starts to burn the calories from stored energy, or fat cells. These fat cells become the only energy source available and therefore are being burned from the body.

This can also happen with one workout while practicing intermittent fasting. During the process of fasting and post-workout, the body does not have enough glucose and glycogen to draw from due to a meal skipped. So instead of burning through carbohydrates, where glucose and glycogen often come from, it is forced to look inward for energy. The easiest energy available is the fat stored in adipose tissue. This helps one to lose weight and become leaner. However, intermittent fasting does not stop there. It also aims to make one more sensitive to insulin. When we eat, our body produces insulin. Many individuals are becoming resistant to insulin because of frequent and short eating intervals on top of the high glycemic index food consumed. The more one eats the more insulin that needs to be produced. While insulin is not inherently bad, if the person is not sensitive enough to insulin, he or she will never feel full and keep eating. Fasting changes how we produce and react to insulin. Due to the lesser amount of food consumed, our body is going to release less insulin. The more insulin sensitive one is, the better the body can store the calories consumed. When one breaks fast and starts eating, the body will either use up that energy immediately, store little of it, or it will be converted to glycogen and stored in muscles for use later. Insulin is what is causing many people to gain weight. This insulin resistance is leading to overweight people and many different diseases. With intermittent fasting reducing insulin fluctuations and production, it creates a bunch of other great benefits.

Chapter 4
Why You Should Embrace
Intermittent Fasting

Contrary to popular belief, Intermittent Fasting is not a new age discovery or 21st-century invention made by scientists studying rats. It is a way of life that has been in existence since time immemorial.

Rather it is an ancient secret, almost like lost history that has only recently been excavated by scientists and so being tested on rats.

To begin with, early man or our predecessors before the age of internet or the age of airplanes and cruise ships, human beings existed and therefore they had to eat because, despite all the modern advancements, the human body pretty much has remained the same, and therefore hunger has been constant. The early man had to go through long periods of fasting due to seasonal variations, drought or famine, and other natural calamities. Even when there were no natural calamities, food was never readily available, and every meal had to be sourced.

If you go back in time and rewind to tales of your parent's childhood or your grandparent's childhood, you will recollect how they never had access to leftover food. They always had fresh, simple meals made with ingredients found in their vicinity. This was the way of life until recently.

Have you wondered how before the advent of supermarkets or before the advent of refrigerators how did people eat? The answer to Intermittent Fasting lies in these questions because, back in the day when there were no refrigerators and supermarkets, the humble human being lived the life of "hunter-gatherer." Living as a hunter-gatherer meant eating when one was able to gather food. When no food was available, they did not eat and yet the human species managed to survive.

The body has a wonderful capacity to store food in the form of fat, and it uses these fat reserves when there is no additional fuel in the form of food being provided continuously without a break.

When the body starts using the fat reserves, there is no accumulation of weight, and therefore there was no concept of "Weight Loss." There was also no accumulation of weight because the early man had to first hunt for every meal because, remember, no refrigerator, which meant a lot of physical activity since there was no neighborhood supermarket where he or she could go to procure food.

Technology and innovation changed the way humans have evolved. Industrialization completely changed the food industry. Factories started mushrooming during industrialization, and this introduced the concept of mass production of food. Mass production of food meant that markets are always flooded with food products. The concept of famine started to fade slowly. After all, humans finally found a way to grow food with or without rainfall. All this changed the way human's view and consume food.

All the physical activity and the lack of access to food continuously meant that the human body would go into "fasting mode" from the "being fed" mode and use up the fat conserved.

Confusing, right? But what do these terms "fasting mode" and "being fed mode," mean? It almost makes your body sound like a machine with various modes to function.

Being fed mode means continuously eating every few hours. This kind of lifestyle has been in vogue for the last few years where people have been encouraged to eat small meals every few hours. If you eat every few hours, your body is in the "fed" mode.

Fasting mode means when a person stops eating and has not fed the body anything for some time. These days the only time a person goes into fasting mode is while they are asleep.

So, from a hunter-gatherer, man has come to a stage now where he or she is constantly in the fed mode. While the body is in the fed mode, it absorbs, digests, and assimilates all the nutrients from the food being fed. In this state, it does not burn any energy or fat because it is constantly working to digest the food. It does not burn any fat because it depends on the nutrients present in the food being fed to provide the energy required for functioning.

Since the body does not burn fat in the fed state, weight loss does not happen. Weight loss only happens when there is a caloric deficit, i.e., only when the body is not being fed and goes into fasting mode. Once the body enters fasting mode, it starts using the reserves of fat that it has stored away, and therefore weight loss happens. During the fasting state, the body burns fat reserves to provide energy for functioning.

Intermittent fasting is a way of life and not a diet. It was the only way of life known to man before the industrial revolution took over society and supermarkets cropped up. Technological advancements have made it possible for fruit and vegetables to grow in all seasons, in all shapes and sizes. Technology has made it possible to store food for months together, and the mushrooming of online markets has made it possible to procure any food with one click and not leaving the confines of home.

But all this has also brought with it major health problems. While technological evolution has happened aggressively, biological evolution has not happened, and human beings have sadly not been able to catch up.

People often confuse "fasting" with "starvation" and use these words interchangeably. Contrary to popular belief, starvation and fasting are very different concepts. Fasting is a conscious decision to skip meals and not eat, despite food being accessible. Starvation is involuntary when you want to eat but cannot because of food not being available and not knowing when the next meal will be available. By fasting and eventually feasting, it helps to consume food only during a specific time of the day and choose not to eat for a larger window of time.

The early man went through both periods of fasting and starvation. Consciously fasting has never killed a human being, whereas you have read about starvation leading to death. In the case of fasting, food is accessible, and the brain knows this. So, there is no sense of fear and insecurity since you know that your next meal is available.

Centuries later, it is this concept that is being repackaged and sold as "Intermittent Fasting" to millions of people.

Intermittent fasting relies on the fundamental concept of moving the state of the body from the "being fed" mode to "fasting mode" and maintaining the fasting mode from anywhere between 8-16 hours.

You would "intermittently" eat during a short window of the day and "fast" during a larger window. Intermittent fasting is not a diet since you are eating!! It is not a starvation diet, but rather a healthy lifestyle. It is a way of living that you could sustain for the rest of your life.

The important word to remember is "fasting." This book will explain in detail:

- How intermittent fasting works

- The benefits of fasting

- The methods of fasting

- The demerits of fasting

To sum it up, intermittent fasting is simple enough that you will do, meaningful enough since it will make a difference.

Chapter 5
How It Works

How Intermittent Fasting Works

How does intermittent fasting work? Well, it takes advantage of the two opposing states in the body and uses them to stipulate when you should eat and when you should avoid food to achieve weight loss. These two states are:

The Fed State

The first state your body can be in is known as the fed state. In this state, you are eating, digesting, and absorbing food. When in the fed state, your body increases insulin production. As a result, fat burning is halted, and your body starts using up the glucose you are providing it with. Any excess calories you consume end up being stored in your fat cells.

The fed state begins when you take the first bite, and it typically lasts for 3-5 hours. Many people constantly find themselves in the fed state because they eat every 3-4 hours. Here is where it gets interesting. Excess calories are stored when you are in the fed state. This means that your body has many opportunities to store calories in the fat cells if you are constantly in the fed state. The more time you spend in the fed state, the greater the chances of weight gain.

To lose weight, you must give your body enough time actually to burn the fat in your fat stores. This is where the fasted state comes in.

The Fasted State

After going through the fed state, your body goes into the post-absorptive stage. In this stage, your body still has access to the components of your last meal. This state lasts for 8-12 hours after you have had your last meal. However, once the 12 hours are up, you will enter the fasted state fully. Many people do not spend time in the fasted state. Once they wake up, they break their fast by eating breakfast, and they enter the fed state all over again. This gives the body all the glucose it needs. If the body has access to glucose, it will not burn fat. Therefore, intermittent fasting is important.

When you adopt intermittent fasting, you will be fasting for at least 16 hours. This gives your body enough time to deplete whatever food components you give it. Once they are depleted, your body will cry out for more fuel. The keyword is fuel.

The fuel your body needs does not have to come from carbohydrates (glucose). In the absence of glucose, your body can effectively turn to fat burning when it needs more energy. Intermittent fasting gives it that option. Once you start burning fat, you will lose weight. Your body will use up the fat in its fat stores simply because you have allowed it to.

Thus, it is important to know when to eat and when to fast. To do this, you will need to determine which intermittent fasting protocol to follow.

Chapter 6
Benefits of Intermittent Fasting

Numerous studies prove and reiterate the multiple benefits of intermittent fasting leveraged by our ancestors knowingly or unknowingly. Intermittent fasting has positive effects both on your body and mind. When you start your regime, you will notice many good things taking place in your body.

Health Benefits

Maintains healthy blood sugar levels

Carbohydrates from the food we eat are broken down into glucose or sugar in our bloodstream. Insulin transports the glucose from our bloodstream to the cells where it is converted into energy. Diabetes is a condition in which insulin does not function effectively, leading to high levels of sugar in the bloodstream along with multiple symptoms such as frequent urination, thirst, and fatigue.

Studies on intermittent fasting eating patterns have proved that it helps in maintaining blood sugar levels by preventing insulin, sugar spikes and crashes leading to reduced risks of diabetes. Other studies were conducted with participants who had diabetes, and the observations from these studies revealed intermittent fasting not only helped in weight loss and controlled calorie intake but also reduced blood sugar levels.

Studies also proved that individuals on intermittent fasting eating patterns showed a 12% decrease in blood sugar level and a 53% reduction in insulin levels. These figures are reflective of the power of intermittent fasting methods in maintaining healthy blood sugar levels. Lowered insulin levels in the bloodstream prevent build-up which, in turn, increases our insulin-sensitivity allowing the critical hormone to work more efficiently.

Improves Heart Health

Intermittent fasting is proven to have a lot of benefits for heart health by lowering the incidences of certain heart-related risk factors or health markers as they are known in medical terminology.

Studies proved that intermittent fasting reduces unhealthy triglycerides and LDL cholesterol levels and increases healthy HDL cholesterol levels. In some intermittent fasting studies on animals, it was observed that adiponectin protein levels improved. This protein involved in the metabolism of sugar and fat is believed to be useful in the prevention of heart attacks and heart disorders.

Intermittent fasting is also known to balance blood pressure levels, another key risk factor for heart problems. Although many of these studies are animal-based, experts are of the opinion that these benefits could be manifested in humans too.

Reduces Inflammation and Oxidative Stress

Although inflammation is nothing but our body's natural immune response to any kind of injury, chronic inflammation can potentially cause health disorders. Some studies have connected chronic inflammation to cancer, heart disease, obesity, and diabetes.

Studies on people who were following the Ramadan fast showed reduced levels of inflammatory-related risk factors. Nighttime fasts were also linked to lowered levels of inflammatory markers. Alternate-day fasting studies revealed lowered risk factors associated with oxidative stress, another marker directly connected to risks of chronic diseases.

Oxidation is a process that involves free radicals, or unstable molecules, to react with and damage healthy and stable molecules such as proteins and DNA. Multiple studies have revealed the usefulness of intermittent fasting to build our resistance to oxidative stress.

Improves Brain Function and Cognitive Abilities and Reduces Neurodegenerative Risks

Most elements that are good for your body are typically good for the brain too, and so it is with intermittent fasting. Intermittent fasting is shown to improve multiple metabolic features critical for the health of your brain and improved cognitive functions.

These metabolic features that get a boost with intermittent fasting include reduced inflammation, oxidative stress, reduced blood sugar levels, and improved insulin sensitivity. Some animal studies have revealed that intermittent fasting can help in the growth of new nerve cells which could have a direct connection to brain function.

Additionally, intermittent fasting is believed to improve levels of brain-derived neurotrophic factor (BDNF), an important brain hormone. BDNF is a protein which interacts with the nerve cells in the basal forebrain, hippocampus, and cortex; all of which are linked to human cognitive functions such as learning and memory.

BDNF is also known to facilitate the survival and growth of existing neurons as well as stimulating the growth of new neurons. It is also connected to the neuro-synaptic connectivity between neurons. The deficiency of this critical brain hormone is connected to depression and other brain-related mental disorders including cognitive impairment, memory loss, and Alzheimer's. Antidepressants increase the level of BDNF, and so does fasting.

Animal studies have also revealed that intermittent fasting could protect the brain from stroke-related damage. Intermittent fasting studies on animals have also revealed that it could delay the onset or reduce the symptoms of neurodegenerative diseases such as Alzheimer's, Huntington's, and Parkinson's.

Healthy Pancreas and Liver

The pancreas is the organ responsible for the production and release of insulin. As your body becomes sensitive to insulin, the pancreas does not get overworked by overproduction of this critical hormone leading to a healthy pancreas.

Intermittent fasting is also known to make your liver healthy by helping it fight against excessive storage of fat. Intermittent fasting produces proteins responsible for the absorption and storage of fatty acids in the liver, thereby freeing it from having to absorb and hold too much fat.

Improved Sensitivity to Hunger Cues

Leptin, a hormone produced by fat cells, is connected to satiety. It sends signals to you to stop eating when satiated. Leptin levels increase when you feel full and decrease when you feel hungry.

As fat cells produce leptin, obese and overweight individuals typically have high levels of leptin in their body. Excessive leptin potentially leads to leptin resistance thereby making it difficult for your body to read and turn off hunger cues when you are feeling full.

Studies conducted on people who were following intermittent fasting revealed lower levels of leptin during the fasting period. Reduced leptin levels typically translate to improved leptin sensitivity, enabling your body to interpret hunger cues well and prevent overeating.

Intermittent fasting helps in correcting eating disorders by enhancing the body's sensitivity to the various hormones. It helps in reversing binge eating and resetting the natural eating pattern of the human body.

Improves Lifespan

Intermittent fasting studies on animals have revealed its ability to extend lifespan. Many studies on rats gave startling results wherein the rats that were on alternate-day fasting lived 83% longer than those animals which were not on any fast.

Other Healthy Changes in Your Body

Improved Productivity and Energy

When we consume excessive foods, especially processed foods, our minds become dull and our energies are at a low level. On the contrary, studies have proven that on an empty stomach, focus and concentration powers improve significantly.

When you fast, the energies that would have been used to digest the consumed food will be channelized for other more productive work including cell repair and regeneration. Additionally, enhanced cognitive powers (a benefit of intermittent fasting) also help in improving alertness, focus, and mental accuracy.

Fasting makes you feel 'light' which gives you an energy boost. Another reason for this boost of energy is that during a normal eating pattern, our energy source is from carbs and sugars which provide 4 calories per gram. When on a fasting pattern, your body draws energy from fats which give 9 calories per gram, thereby boosting our natural energy levels.

Improved Skin Texture

Oxidative stress from free radicals and chronic inflammation can damage and cause your skin to wrinkle up and form fine lines as well. Intermittent fasting reduces both oxidative stress and inflammation resulting in improved and smooth skin texture. Intermittent fasting helps clear your skin of acne and pimples, giving it a glowing, vibrant look.

Improved Lean Mass

During any weight loss program, you would typically lose both muscle and fat. Losing fat is great but losing muscle is not. Intermittent fasting speeds up fat metabolism, resulting in more fat loss and insignificant lean mass loss.

Flatter belly

When the body turns to fat for its fuel, it succeeds in breaking down and releasing energy from stubborn belly fat too. Therefore, a sustained effort at intermittent fasting is bound to help you achieve a flatter belly than before.

Improved Motor Skills

Motor abilities such as balance can be affected significantly with aging. There are multiple studies which prove that improved fasting helps in decreasing the effects of motor disabilities associated with aging.

Improved Sleep

Research has proven that intermittent fasting can improve sleeping patterns and can reset your sleeping pattern if it has been disturbed by travel.

Improved Sensitivity to Taste

Getting addicted to excessively sugary, salty, and processed foods is easy. However, the overwhelming tastes from these types of foods lower our taste buds' sensitivity. The taste buds forget how to appreciate and savor wholesome, earthy, and healthy flavors.

After a fasting period, your taste buds are reset to the original natural state, and these grainy and earthy flavors become delicious again. Moreover, as you sustain your fasting efforts, you will notice that you will lessen the amounts of sugars and salts in your food to savor their taste. Even the subtlest of flavors are easily discernible by your sensitive taste buds.

Psychological Benefits

In addition to physical and other health benefits that fasting offers, there is a multitude of psychological benefits you can take advantage of when you choose the intermittent fasting way of staying healthy and fit. Let's explore some of these psychological benefits.

Improved Willpower

Sabotaging behaviors, destructive addictions, and giving in to your desires without a fight are all examples of the opposite of willpower. All these elements slowly but surely ruin your life and relationships. Bad decisions taken because of the lack of willpower will weaken you even further and stunt your growth and development.

If you continue to justify your poor decisions because of your weak willpower, you are only adding fuel to the fire, creating irreparable bad habits for life. Bad habits reflect your inability to control yourself, and if you cannot control yourself, you can hardly control anything else.

Fasting is a natural way of learning to control your responses and reactions to your physical needs and desires. When you fast, you are voluntarily choosing not to eat, even under the pressure of hunger pangs. You are choosing to fast (give up food) to gain something else (health and fitness).

Food is the most basic element of survival and eating when hungry is the fundamental survival instinct. Therefore, when you control this basic survival instinct by choosing not to eat even when you feel hungry, you will find your willpower increasing in strength. You will find the power to control other less fundamental and yet, debilitating bad habits that are ruining your life.

Fasting is the most natural and the most sophisticated form of workout to build your willpower. If you develop the habit of fasting, you will be able to control many other debilitating habits of your life more efficiently. There are medical studies which prove that fasting can dissipate cravings for alcohol, nicotine, caffeine, etc.

So, build and strengthen your willpower by making intermittent fasting a habit in your life.

Improves Self-Confidence

Self-control is the foundation of self-confidence. Confidence is nothing but a reflection of your ability for self-control. So, when you lose self-control, you are effectively sabotaging your self-confidence. The reverse is also true. When you build your self-control, you build and strengthen your self-confidence.

Lack of self-confidence causes plenty of internal conflicts which have the debilitating power of corroding your willpower. These unceasing internal conflicts leave you exhausted and on a perpetual defensive mode resulting in further reduction in self-confidence.

Now, suppose you build your self-control and behave the way you always intended to behave. The results of these intended actions will build your self-confidence as you develop greater trust in your capabilities and strengths. With each success, you will find the power to take on more challenging goals and tasks and eventually build your self-efficacy to such an extent that you are in complete control of your future and destiny.

Fasting is the most effective way to practice self-control and, consequently, build self-confidence. Medical studies have also revealed that fasting improves catecholamines in your body. Catecholamines (for example, dopamine) are believed to be connected to your happiness, confidence, and feel-good emotions and also reduce anxiety and stress levels.

Improved Clarity of Thought

With enhanced brain functioning and cognitive powers, your ability to think clearly will improve. Eating dulls your thoughts and fasting creates clarity. When you fast, your brain and body can catch even subtle signals, and you can see the things going wrong in your life.

While fasting, you can very quickly notice the incongruent elements in your life such as bad habits, poor organization, lack of purpose and intention, and more. This clear perspective is bound to make you take corrective steps.

With improved willpower and self-confidence, you will find the necessary physical and mental strength to overcome challenges and improve the overall quality of your life. Fasting can be a great resetting mode for the psychological aspect of your life.

Improved Emotions

Excessive eating is effectively an emotional dependency. Foods such as processed sugars, caffeine, and trans-fatty acids, and alcohol are all known to over-stimulate our emotions and, therefore, abstaining from eating occasionally helps in stabilizing our emotions.

Fasting can also reset your negative emotion pattern, and you can break free of their harmful effects. Moreover, fasting helps us have a different perceptive of our environment, enhancing our clarity to see what and how things are going wrong in our lives. Such sharp perceptions automatically drive us to reshape our environments for improved quality of life.

The sustained efforts of intermittent fasting can have startling benefits for you. Each one of the benefits mentioned in this chapter is possible. Some of them may manifest faster than others. Patience, perseverance, and commitment are vital elements to leverage nearly all the benefits of intermittent fasting.

Chapter 7
Intermittent Fasting Methods

The good thing about an intermittent fast is that you get a choice in the kind you want to go on. There are a few options you can choose to go with depending on how long you want to fast, and which one ends up working the best for your schedule. You may find that one is easier for you to implement, and others seem to give you better results than others. This chapter is going to look at some of the different types of intermittent fasts that you can consider using to help you get the amazing results that you want!

The 16/8 Method

A popular method that you can use when it comes to intermittent fasting is the 16/8 method. This is when you will fast each day for a total of 14 to 16 hours, and then you will restrict your eating window for that day to only 8 to 10 hours. When you are in your eating window, you will fit in two or three meals. This helps you to limit the amount of time that you are eating each day, which can naturally cut down on the calories that you consume.

This method is a popular one to follow because it simply could mean not having anything to eat after you finish dinner and then skipping breakfast or moving breakfast back a few hours. So, if you complete your last meal at 6 pm and don't take a snack or anything after dinner, you could start eating the next day by 10 am, enjoying a late breakfast or an early lunch.

Women who want to go with this type of intermittent fasting should try not to fast for more than sixteen hours. This seems to work better with the hormones and natural rhythm for women and is safer for them to keep up with.

During this type of fast, you can drink coffee, water, and other non-caloric beverages to help you reduce the hunger that you feel. And when it comes to the eating window, you need to make sure that you eat a healthy diet rather than a lot of junk or too many calories. This makes it easier to maintain the fast and can help you to lose weight. In the beginning, you may have some hunger pains as you get used to not being able to eat the second you wake up in the morning, but overall, this is an easy method of intermittent fasting to follow.

The 5:2 Diet

Another popular version of the intermittent fasting diet is known as the 5:2 diet. This one involves the individual eating a normal diet for 5 days of the week. Then they will pick two days of the week where they will keep their calories to between 500 and 600. You can pick the two days that you want to fast on, but try to not have them right by each other, or you may run into troubles with not consuming too much when it's time to eat again.

On these fasting days, you would keep your calories to about 500 for the whole day. Try to get in as many nutrients as possible, but you can also catch up a bit when you get done with the fasting period. Most people split their day into two 250 calorie meals to help them get through this day. But if you are worried about overeating, it may be best to go the day without eating, and then have one 500 calorie meal.

The Eat Stop Eat Method

The eat stop eat method is going to involve doing a 24 hour fast, usually one or two times each week. As long as you don't do the fasting for two days in a row. So, you might pick Tuesday and Friday as your fasting days. This method doesn't have to be as difficult as it seems. You could stop eating after supper one day and then eat at dinner the next day. This method can ensure that you aren't going to bed hungry each night. Or you can change it up to work with what is best for your schedule. If you want to go from breakfast one day to breakfast the next, or lunch one day to lunch the next, that is fine as well.

During this fast, you can have coffee, water, and any other non-caloric beverages. But you can't eat any solid food during this time. This can be hard to do, but it can give you some amazing results if you can keep it up. Pick a day when you are going to be busy anyway and would have a lot of trouble getting to a meal, and then this won't be as hard.

If you choose the eat stop eat method to help you lose weight, then you need to make sure that during your eating windows, you eat as normally as you can. Try to eat the same amount of food as you would if you didn't fast. Don't overeat when it is time to start eating again. This helps to even you out to fewer calories through the week, and you will lose weight.

Some beginners find that going with the eat stop eat method can be hard. They will feel hungry, and they may have trouble making it through the whole day. If you haven't ever done an intermittent fast before, then consider doing one of the smaller fasts first, such as a fast for 16 hours. Get used to this and then move up to the eat stop eat method.

Alternate Day Fasting

With an alternate day fast, you are going to need to fast every other day. You will take one day where you can eat like normal and then the other day needs to be some kind of fast. There are variations on this. Some will ask you not to eat anything during your fasting day, and others will allow you to have around 500 calories during your fasting days.

If you have read any studies on intermittent fasting, including some that are included in this guidebook, the intermittent fasting method they discuss is alternate day fasting. This one can give you a lot of health benefits, but for a beginner, a full day of fasting every other day of the week can be hard. This method is going to leave you feeling hungry several times a week, which can be unpleasant. Starting with a different option can often be the best way to get used to fasting before moving onto this one.

The Warrior Diet

Another option that you can choose is known as the Warrior Diet, and this one is often considered the most difficult to follow, simply because the eating window is often small. It can be hard to keep yourself from eating most of the day, and it is even harder to get enough nutrients into your day in such a short period as well.

The Warrior diet is going to involve eating small amounts of vegetables and fruits, raw if possible, during the day. The amount that you take in should only add up to a few hundred calories in total. Then you can have one large meal at night. You are going to be on a fast all day long and then have a feast at night with a four-hour eating window.

The Warrior diet is one of the first popular types of diets that used the idea of intermittent fasting to help. In addition to worrying about such a strict eating window, this diet is going to emphasize food choices that are very similar to being on the Paleo diet. This means that you need to eat foods that are whole, unprocessed, and ones that look like they do in nature.

Spontaneous Meal Skipping

Some people don't want to be on a regular intermittent fast. They don't want to be tied down to something all the time, or maybe they worry about what going on a strict fast would do to their system. But they recognize that it is better for them to listen to their bodies and not just eat non-stop each day. These individuals may choose to go with the process of spontaneous meal skipping or skipping out on meals when it is convenient for them, rather than following a strict schedule.

Any time that you are too busy to cook and sit down to eat, or any time that you don't feel hungry, you would skip a meal. It is a myth that people have to get something into their stomachs every few hours or they are going to lose a lot of muscle, or they will hit starvation mode. But think about times when you got sick and didn't feel well. You may have gone a few days without eating while you got over an upset stomach, and your metabolism was just fine when you were done.

This is because the human body is set up to handle going longer periods when there isn't food. Unlike modern times, there were often periods when the body would have to go without food during a famine. Missing a few meals on occasion is not going to be that big of a deal to a body that knows how to prepare for the famine.

So, if you feel that you are not hungry at breakfast time one day, you can skip that meal and eat dinner and lunch that is healthier. Or, if you are on the road and can't find something that is healthy to eat, go ahead and do a short fast during that time. This isn't the most stringent of intermittent fasts, but it can provide you with some of the benefits that you get from the other options. What is important here is that you must make sure the other meals are healthy and nutrient dense to get the best benefits.

These are just a few of the options that you can choose from when it comes to going on an intermittent fast. There are also variations on each of these that you can choose to work with. All of them can be effective, although the alternate day fasting is the method that is often cited in studies about this type of eating plan. You need to pick the method that works best for your lifestyle and the one that helps you reach your goals the best.

Chapter 8
Who Should Avoid Fasting

Fasting may be beneficial for most people. Unfortunately, it may not be a one size fits all type of program. While it boasts many different health benefits, some people may not be suited for fasting. Fasting can harm some individuals so always check to make sure you do not have any underlying medical conditions before fasting.

Medical Conditions

Individuals who are not healthy in a mental or physical aspect should not try fasting. If you find that you have a lot of mental stressors in your life, put fasting on the back burner. This does not mean you couldn't plan to engage intermittent fasting later, but until your mind is ready, it's best to skip fasting. If in doubt, always check with your doctor for clearance.

Highly Intensive Workouts

If you have any risk of being frail or malnourished, fasting won't be beneficial for you. This also goes to say that if you are exercising intensively every day, fasting might not be suitable for you. You may still proceed, but special efforts must be made to plan your meal macronutrients and micronutrients intake to ensure you are sufficiently nourished and energy well replenished.

Pregnancy and Breastfeeding

While there is conflicting information out there, pregnant and breastfeeding women should try to avoid regular fasting. Occasionally fasting will not hurt, but intermittent fasting, can affect your nutrients intake for your baby or lower your milk supply. Once you have delivered and stopped breastfeeding, you can benefit better from intermittent fasting.

Diabetics

People with diabetes should also be wary of fasting. While people with type two diabetes may benefit from fasting, it can be very dangerous for a person with type one diabetes. If your diet is currently insulin controlled, do not start fasting unless you have discussed with your medical provider. Fasting can lead to weight loss and stabilization of insulin, which could help type two diabetics, but you need to be aware of how it could affect your insulin in a controlled diet. It is critical to consult professional medical advice before proceeding.

High Cortisol

If you are stressed or dealing with high levels of cortisol in your body, you should not fast. Whether you are monitoring your cortisol levels professionally or just noticing the extra stomach fat, combined with your high-stress levels, it's best to clear yourself from the condition before fasting. Fasting raises your cortisol levels. While this is fine in people with normal cortisol levels, if you are already high on cortisol, this can lead to more weight gain and added stress.

Children

Also, children should not fast. Intermittent fasting is great for adults, but children need proper nutrition intake throughout the day to help their growing bodies.

Other Medical Conditions

Other disorders like kidney disease, anemia, frequent fainting, and liver disease are all other important reasons to avoid fasting. Check with your doctor if you have one of these diseases.

And finally, if you have any history of disordered eating, fasting should be avoided completely. Because of the mental stress fasting can cause, it's recommended that anyone who previously has had an eating disorder should abstain from fasting.

While most people can safely fast, always take notice of your medical conditions and ask your doctor if fasting is best for you.

Chapter 9
What to Eat

It is important to know the type of food to eat during fasting and what foods to avoid during this time. Here is what you should take:

Water

This is the most important element to consume when you take up the intermittent fast. Water can act as an elixir when it comes to losing weight. You must keep your body hydrated and ensure that all the toxins are dissolved and eliminated. All your organs need water to remain fresh and healthy; right from your liver to gut to the digestive tract, water helps to keep these organs working smoothly. Drink at least 8 to 10 glasses of water a day and focus more on the fasting period. It is obvious that it will get a little monotonous, and so, a good idea is to consume fruit-infused water. This refers to water that has fruit and herbs infused into it. Fill up a jar with water and toss in fruit and herbs such as oranges, lemons, mint leaves, and a dash of cinnamon. Consume this every few hours. Remember that the intermittent fast can be quite taxing at times and lead to side effects such as headaches and nausea. In such a case, only water can help you out and put an end to these.

Fish

Fish can be considered a miracle food as it can greatly help with weight loss. According to dietary guidelines, it is important for people to consume at least 6 to 8 ounces of fish every week. Fish contains a lot of nutrients. It is rich in fats and proteins. It is also rich in vitamin D., and this means you do not have to worry about denying your body these nutrients by taking on the fast. You do not have to reach for supplements if you can consume fish regularly. Fish is also rich in DHA, which helps in brain development. You will see that your mind is fresher, and you can think better. Your productivity will increase, and stress will be curbed.

Avocado

You might wonder why avocado is on this list considering it is one of the fattiest foods out there. However, you must understand that the fasting phase can take a toll on your body and so you must consume foods that can keep you going. Avocado is rich in mono-unsaturated fat, which is great for those who tend to get hungry quite fast. It keeps you feeling fuller for longer. You will not find yourself reaching out to eat a snack. Avocado is quite versatile and can be added to your breakfast or lunch menu. Those who tend to include it in their breakfast menu are generally able to go without food for longer periods without complaining about hunger.

Leafy greens

If there is one type of vegetable that we remember being told to consume by our parents, then it must be leafy green vegetables. As we know, leafy green vegetables are loaded with multiple nutrients that are great for your body. These include the likes of kale, broccoli, lettuce, etc. These are loaded with fiber. Fiber, as you know, keeps your body going when you suffer from digestive issues such as constipation. You are sure to go through it when you adopt the intermittent fast. In such a case, it becomes that much more important to consume these vegetables to keep your stomach in good shape. Fiber also makes you feel fuller and not feel too hungry between meals.

Potatoes

The goal is to consume foods that are filling and can keep you going for hours, one such being potatoes. Potatoes are rich in carbs that can keep you sated for hours. Make sure you either steam and mash them or roast them without the addition of any oil or fat. Deep frying them is never an option. Try to consume them with their skin on as the skin contains a lot of nutrition.

Probiotics

When it comes to digestion, both your liver and gut play a very important role. Both need a healthy dose of probiotics to function optimally. If you have an unhealthy gut, then you might suffer from side effects such as constipation and even leaky gut syndrome. One of the best ways to combat these is by consuming as many probiotics as possible. Some natural foods rich in probiotics include kombucha and kefir. Add these to your meals, and you are sure to experience positive benefits. An alternative is to go for probiotic supplements. Make sure you know which ones to go for. It would be best consulting a physician first.

Assorted berries

There is nothing better than consuming fresh berries in the mornings. They are loaded with antioxidants and vital nutrients required to keep your body healthy. Strawberries, raspberries, blueberries, and gooseberries all are great for you. Just toss them into the blender with some milk or yogurt to make a smoothie. According to studies, those who consumed berries regularly were able to remain within their ideal body weight and did not gain too much weight over long periods.

Eggs

An important aspect of losing weight is building lean muscles. Lean muscles replace regular ones and prevent fat from getting stored. The best way to build lean muscle is by consuming foods rich in proteins. One important source of proteins are eggs. Those who consume eggs for breakfast are in a better position to develop lean muscles and not go hungry before the next meal. Eggs can be quite versatile and cooked in any way you like. Hard-boil them the previous day so that you have a ready meal the next morning. Simply toss them in a pan to scramble them. It only takes a few minutes to cook them.

Whole grains

One aspect of maintaining a clean and healthy diet is going for whole grains. The intermittent fast promotes consumption of these, as they are easier for the body to digest and keep the system clean. They are also loaded with proteins and fiber. Do not limit yourself to the usual, such as wheat and oats, and go for something different such as Bulgar, amaranth, and flax.

Legumes

If you wish to remain full for longer and not feel hungry or peckish too often, then there is nothing better than legumes and beans. These cannot only be quite flavorful but are also loaded with fiber. The body does not easily digest fiber. The body cannot digest it at all but makes an extra effort in trying to digest it thereby drawing into the fat reserves. It is, therefore, best to load up on fiber to lose weight easily. There are many options to pick from including peas, lentils, green beans, fava, black-eyed peas, etc. These easily fit into soups and salads.

Nuts

Nuts are fatty, no doubt, but they contain good fat. Not all fat is bad fat as there can be some good fat as well. Polyunsaturated fats are said to be good for the body and can keep you feeling fuller for longer. You will not feel hungry if you munch on some walnuts or almonds. But make sure you make them a part of your meal and do not snack on them. Snacking on them can leave you feeling full and disrupt your meal plan. Do not worry about the calorie aspect. Nuts are not as calorific as you may think. They contain far fewer calories than some of the other fatty foods that people tend to snack on.

These happen to be superfoods that you must include in your diet while you take up intermittent fasting.

Chapter 10
What to Avoid

When eating to reduce inflammation, it is best to avoid most packaged foods because they contain inflammation-triggering preservatives, colorings, and artificial flavorings to increase their shelf life. If it is packaged in a box or bag, the chances are that it's not good for your health. Eating too many inflammatory foods can lead to chronic low-grade inflammation, which in turn can cause serious health issues including cancer, heart disease, diabetes, and allergies. With that said, this chapter looks at seven specific inflammatory foods to avoid.

Gluten and Wheat

Inflammation is the natural response of your immune system. When we get a splinter, inflammation makes the surrounding area red and tender. With this picture in mind, let's look at why you should avoid gluten.

Proteins found in wheat are gut irritants, and the term "gluten" is a general name for these proteins. Now, picture tiny splinters raking into the lining of your gut and resulting in inflammation. When it comes to gluten, the most well-known gluten-related inflammation is celiac disease or non-celiac gluten sensitivity, but wheat can also be a problem for people who aren't specifically sensitive to gluten because of amylase trypsin inhibitors (ATIs) found in wheat. These ATIs can bring about an inflammatory immune response in the GI tract which contributes to another problem called intestinal permeability, or leaky gut. This condition lets undigested food particles, bacteria, and toxic waste products "leak" through the intestines into your bloodstream.

Refined Carbohydrates

Carbohydrates are commonly referred to as "good" and "bad." Complex carbs are good because they are filled with beneficial fiber. When it comes to inflammation, refined carbohydrates fall into the bad category because in the refining process most of their fiber is removed. With the fiber removed, refined carbs raise blood sugar levels and raise the occurrence of inflammatory changes. This influence can lead to disease. For instance, when looking at our modern diet, research has shown refined carbs can encourage the development of inflammatory bacteria in the gut which can raise the probability of obesity and IBS.

Milk Lactose

Milk lactose is a sugar found in milk which causes digestive issues for many people because their bodies don't produce the lactase enzyme required to digest it. Other people who do produce this enzyme may still react poorly to drinking milk because of the proteins casein and whey. Casein has a molecular structure very similar to gluten, and half the people who can't tolerate gluten don't tolerate casein well either. As a result, dairy is one of the most inflammatory foods in today's diet, second only to gluten. Adverse digestive symptoms resulting from this inflammation may manifest in bloating, constipation, diarrhea, and gas. Other non-digestive symptoms include acne and a compelling demonstration of autistic behaviors. So, lactose is only half the issue when it comes to milk and milk products; the others are the casein and whey proteins.

A study also showed that women in China have a far lower rate of breast cancer than women in the West. The only noticeable difference between the two diets is lower milk intake. A Harvard professor has also discovered links between ovarian cancer and dairy consumption.

Sugar

It's no secret that eating too many added sugars and refined carbohydrates can lead to obesity, but the consequences of eating excesses are also linked to increased gut permeability, raised inflammatory markers, and high LDL cholesterol. The thing all these factors have in common is that they can trigger low-grade chronic inflammation. Excess body fat, especially belly fat, results in continuous, chronic levels of inflammation, which can modify how insulin works. Insulin, as a regulatory hormone, plays a big part in carrying the glucose in your bloodstream into your cells for energy, but when blood glucose levels are chronically high, the production and regulation of insulin is changed, resulting in insulin resistance. The resulting overabundance of blood glucose can lead to an accumulation of advanced glycation end products (AGEs). When too many AGEs bind with our cells and integral proteins, it can lead to oxidative stress and inflammation. It can change their structure, inhibit their regular function, and eventually result in a buildup of arterial plaque and decreased kidney function, amongst other things.

Meat

Grain-fed beef has been touted as tasting better, but cows are naturally grazers that eat grass. When fed grain they grow fat quickly before they are sold by the pound for profit. Cattle, pigs, and chickens are not naturally grain eaters. But in life on the feed-lot, not only are they fed things like corn and soy, but they are also given antibiotics to make sure they don't get sick. This translates to meats on our dinner table that are not only higher in inflammatory saturated fats but also contain higher levels of inflammatory omega-6s from their unnatural diet. To compound the problem, when we grill our meat at high temperatures, it results in inflammatory carcinogens! So, if you plan to eat meat, choose grass-fed varieties.

Saturated Fats

When you think saturated fats, many people think of red meat, but aside from fatty cuts of beef, saturated fat is also found in pork and lamb, the skin of a chicken, as well as processed meats. It's also found in dairy products like butter, cream (including whipped cream), cheese, and regular-fat milk. Studies have linked the consumption of saturated fats with causing the kind of body fat that stores energy rather than burns it. As these fat cells grow bigger; they release pro-inflammatory drivers that promote systemic inflammation.

Alcohol

Drinking alcohol puts a burden on the liver, and when consumed in excess, it weakens liver function. This disrupts other multi-organ interactions resulting in inflammation. If you choose to drink alcohol, do so in moderation, but it is best eliminated if you're fighting inflammation.

Chapter 11
IF for weight loss

It is obvious that our bodies go through different reactions when we consume food and go on a fast. When a person eats, their body requires a little time to process the food and digest it. It does its best to burn away as much as it can. Once it is done, the remainder is stored as fat. The amount of fat depends on the type of meal you have eaten.

On the other hand, when you take up intermittent fasting, you put your body in a position where it readily draws from the available fat reserves. This makes it easier for you to lose excess weight and keep it from adding back on.

You can condition your body to think and act a certain way. It will be easier for your body to burn away whatever is available in the bloodstream. If you have had a sugary meal, then the body will have to put in a lot of effort to spend it all. It would not be able to do so unless you got on a treadmill for an hour just after the meal.

The body must burn carbs to supply fuel to carry out daily activities. If you keep supplying your body with this energy, then it will never resort to drawing it out from the fat reserves.

So, when you fast, you deny your body any easy carbs to burn as fuel. This forces it to dig deep into the reserves and draw them out to burn as fuel. There will be no readily available glucose in your bloodstream, which makes it ideal for weight loss to set in. So, this burning fat results in weight loss.

Having said all that, do not expect to lose weight within a month. Although the process sounds quite simple, it can be a complicated process. Do not assume that you will start losing weight just by not eating food for a few hours. It requires systematic planning and execution. Intermittent fasting is not a fad or yo-yo diet. It is lifestyle modification.

You might be a little taken aback by how slow it goes at the beginning. But you will be surprised at the level at which you will begin to lose fat and develop leaner muscle. You will feel your body shrinking and be able to get into smaller clothes. In fact, you will be able to show off your curves and contours and further boost your confidence to get into fasting on a more serious note.

Although the intermittent fast is designed to help you lose weight without indulging in physical exercise, it is always advisable to do some. Not only will it help you tone down more but also eliminate the melted fat in your body. The body will find it easier to draw from the reserves. All you must do is provide enough energy to your body to carry out the exercises. There is a plethora of choices when it comes to exercises. You can go for skipping, running, swimming, gym, etc.

Insulin

I'm sure you have heard about insulin. Most people associate it with diabetes and how insulin dysfunction can lead to it. When we consume food, our body automatically produces insulin. The faster your body can use this insulin, the better the results. This means that your body will be able to better break down the consumed food depending on how fast it absorbs the insulin and puts it to work. This can offset weight loss much faster and make you lose weight easily. In fact, it can lead to the creation of leaner muscle that will replace the fat cells.

When you fast, you increase insulin sensitivity. Your body becomes that much more sensitive to insulin release and absorption. This means that it goes after the existing glucose in your body that is stored as fat. It draws energy from this glucose to supply your body with fuel.

You must acquaint yourself with the concept of glycogen. It refers to starch that is present in your liver and muscles. Your body tends to turn to it in case it needs energy. However, in most cases, it ends up being dissipated when you start fasting. If you can get your body to bring down its levels by working out regularly, then it will further increase your insulin sensitivity.

This implies that physical activity automatically makes it easier for the body to draw from reserves and use it to up the insulin availability. Food that is stored as glycogen will be burned away to supply energy.

So, plan out your exercise regime in such a way that you take up a rigorous routine right after a heavy meal. Since you are most likely going to consume a heavy breakfast, it would be best to go for an exercise routine about 2 hours after breakfast. Keep it light and fun. If you go for a rigorous routine, then you will end up losing interest in it, as it will be too taxing. Try out new workouts such as Zumba or go for belly dancing. Not only will you lose weight but also thoroughly enjoy yourself. Don't worry if you feel like you do not have the body or moves for it; you are not doing it to enter a competition.

Just make sure you have fun and do not think of it as an arduous task. It always helps to have company. Ask someone to join in so that it does not get too awkward and you remain motivated to persist with it. With time, you will realize that you are automatically getting better at it and can use it to your advantage.

Now imagine adopting this lifestyle and compare it with what you currently have. Weight loss is not easy and requires a lot of effort from your end. On a normal day, you would have consumed 5 meals and had no exercise. It is obvious that your glycogen levels will be super high. These will not get used up at all and will get stored as fat. You must give your body enough means to get rid of the fat reserves.

You might have noticed that most diabetic patients are overweight. This is because they will have a lot of glucose in their body that is not used up fully. This leads to insulin dysfunction. It is therefore important to be well within your ideal BMI and make sure you remain within your ideal weight range.

HGH

Apart from insulin, there is another hormone that is known to help induce weight loss and keep it off. Known as the human growth hormone or HGH, it is one that helps strengthen muscle power. As we know, muscles are very important, and one must try to build lean muscle.

HGH helps to enhance exercise performance. Your body will be in a better position to fulfill exercise routines. Those who are obese tend to have lower levels of response to this hormone's stimuli. HGH aides to offset lipolysis, which refers to the breaking down of lipids or fat reserves in the body.

According to a study, obese people who were put on a diet and given HGH were able to increase their weight loss by almost double compared to those who were not put on it. The best part of the experiment was that they were able to reduce visceral fat, which happens to be one of the toughest forms of fat to fight away. In the group that did not receive HGH, it was found that they had lost out on lean body mass. But with the group that received the hormones, their lean body mass had increased.

This shows that HGH is great when it comes to losing weight holistically. When you fast, this hormone automatically increases.

This hormone is consistently produced and secreted all through the day and night. You do not have to do anything, as the fast will take care of it.

HGH in combination with an increase in insulin sensitivity will end up making weight loss that much easier. Your body will be ready for lean muscle growth.

To put it simply, intermittent fasting tells your body the best way in which the food you consume can be used. It makes sure your body knows that the food is being supplied so that it can start the process of digging into the fat reserve and use it as fuel. This automatically offsets weight loss.

Treat every meal as a celebratory meal and enjoy it. Do not be in a hurry to eat something and rush to your next job. Make it a point to sit down and savor the meal. Spend at least 30 minutes understanding all the flavors involved, the textures involved, etc.

Chapter 12
How to Get Started

Well, now that you know what Intermittent Fasting is all about and how it works, the next step is for you to get started with this diet. Intermittent Fasting is not merely a dieting protocol, but a way of life. Intermittent Fasting is sustainable in the long run and isn't a short-term diet. If you want to achieve and maintain your weight loss and overall health, then you must stick to this diet. Intermittent Fasting will help you shed all those extra kilos you want to lose. In this section, you will learn about the different steps that you can follow to get started on this diet.

Starting a new diet might seem slightly intimidating, but with the help of these steps, it will not seem intimidating.

Step 1: Select a Method

There are various Intermittent Fasting protocols that you can choose from. One of the most versatile patterns of dieting these days is Intermittent Fasting. You need to opt for a method that fits your lifestyle, personality, and meets your goals. If you are used to waking up early and like exercising, then the method of Intermittent Fasting that you can opt for is the 16:8 method. If you choose this method, then you can have breakfast in the morning and have your last meal in the evening. If you are used to skipping breakfast or don't mind skipping breakfast, then you can have your first meal at noon and your last meal at night. If you don't like the idea of fasting days, then you can choose the alternate day fasting protocol and fast on alternate days. The method that you opt for is entirely up to you. You can customize this diet to meet your requirements. There is a method of fasting that will meet your requirements, and you merely need to make up your mind about the method you want to opt for.

Step 2: Research

Go through all the information that is given in this book before you decide to select a specific method. Always select a method that suits your lifestyle. If you do this, it will be quite easy to stick to your dieting protocol. When compared to other conventional diets, this method is quite relaxed, since Intermittent Fasting doesn't place much emphasis on what you eat but instead concentrates on when you eat. Check your priorities and find a method that will suit your needs. Once you establish your goals, you need to research the fasting protocol you want to opt for. If you want to lose fat and gain lean muscle, then the method you must opt for is LeanGains.

Step 3: Find the necessary tools

There are various apps that you can use to help you with this diet. You can choose from free as well as paid applications to track your progress. Intermittent Fasting is essentially a method of trial and error. One method might be quite effective for some while something else might work for others. You can download an application that will help track your progress and determine whether a specific method is effective or not. If you want to, you can also maintain a food journal to track your progress. You need to make a note of when you eat and what you eat, along with the progress you are making.

Step 4: Starting the transition

Starting this diet might be a little tricky if you don't have an all or nothing attitude. If you are used to skipping meals now and then, then Intermittent Fasting will be quite simple. If you are not used to fasting and have never fasted before, then it will be a little difficult until you gain some footing. You need to prepare yourself mentally for the diet you want to follow. It might seem a little daunting that you need to go for prolonged periods without eating. Well, the one thing that you need to remember is that all your fears are baseless, and, in fact, there is nothing that you need to fear. The fear is in your head, and you will not get over it unless you take the first step.

You need to take some time to condition your body. To condition your body, you can slowly start increasing the gap between two meals. After you do this, you can start by slowly skipping a meal a day so that your body gets used to the idea of fasting. If you are used to snacking between meals, then you can slowly cut down on snacks. Instead, you can start filling yourself up with foods that will leave you feeling fuller for longer. After you do this, you can start with a relatively easy method of fasting. You can start with the alternate-day fasting method or the LeanGains method. It is all about slowly conditioning yourself to the diet and the idea of dieting. Once you do this, you will be able to follow the diet rather easily.

Step 5: Finding the necessary support

Everyone needs a support system. Your support system will encourage you and motivate you to keep going even when you feel like giving up. You can also start your diet with a diet buddy or partner. Find a partner for yourself and start the diet together. Your dieting buddy can be your partner, spouse, friend, or anyone else. You can each use the other as a coach and a mentor along the way. If you cannot find someone to do this with, then you can explain your situation to someone and make them hold you accountable for the progress you make. Make that person check on you and the progress you are making.

Step 6: Toning down your workouts

You need to tone down your workout routine, at least initially. You need to give your body some time to get used to the new diet before you can go back to your exercise routine. When your body is getting used to a new diet, it is quite likely that you might feel a little low on energy. In such situations, if you push yourself too hard, you risk burning yourself out, and it will not do you any good.

Step 7: Following delayed gratification

Delayed gratification is a brilliant technique, and it works rather well with this form of dieting. There might be times when a hunger pang strikes you, and you might start craving for something sweet. Whenever this happens, make a list of the things that you want to eat. Keep adding items to this list whenever you feel hungry. When this happens, you need to tell yourself that you cannot eat that right now and you can eat it later. When you do this, it helps to stop your mind from obsessing over things that you must not eat. You need to control your mind, and you must not let it control you. You need to eat only those foods that are good for you.

Step 8: Protein must be a Priority

Always make sure that you eat the necessary proteins and complex carbs before anything else. You might have something sweet or oily on your eating list, but all that can wait. If you give in to your urge to eat something you aren't supposed to, then you will end up overeating. Also, it is quite likely that you will fill yourself up with junk during the eating window and then experience hunger pangs when you start fasting. When you are eating, you need to understand that you are prepping your body for the fasting period. So, you must always eat those foods that will leave you feeling fuller for longer like proteins, healthy carbs, and dietary fats.

If you start feeling hungry while fasting, it is likely that you will give up on your diet. To avoid this, eat healthy and wholesome meals.

Avoid all sorts of processed foods that are full of sugars, unhealthy fats, and undesirable carbs. Instead, opt for healthy foods that are rich in fiber, nutrients, and essential macros. Healthy food will nourish your body and will leave you feeling energetic. Unhealthy foods like chocolates or chips can be replaced with some fruits or nuts. Here are a couple of simple tips that you can keep in mind to make sure that you are eating wholesome food.

Have complex carbohydrates like whole grains and leafy vegetables instead of starchy foods like bread, pasta, or pizza. Your meal must be rich in protein because it not only leaves you feeling fuller for longer, but it is good for you as well. Stay away from all processed foods and opt for healthy treats like kale chips, nuts, fruits, or anything that isn't full of saturated fats and trans fats. Replace sugary drinks with water (sparkling or still). Create a food plan for yourself. If you are interested in cooking, then learn to experiment with recipes and cook something different. Healthy food doesn't mean bland salads, so keep an open mind and try your hand at cooking. If you plan your meals in advance, then you can do all the meal prep on your day off, this does simplify the entire cooking process.

Step 9: Taking a "before" photograph

Before you start following any of the protocols of Intermittent Fasting, there is one little step along the way that you need to take. You need to take a photograph of yourself. You can label it as a "before" photograph. This will help you to get started. If you follow the protocols of Intermittent Fasting properly, then you will be able to see a positive change in your body. Keep taking a weekly photograph of yourself and make a timeline of the photographs. It will help you see the progress you are making. At times, you might need a little extra motivation to keep going. Whenever you hit a snag, you simply need to look at your timeline, and it will provide you with the necessary motivation to keep going. Also, keep a track of your body measurements. At times, you might not notice any weight loss, but you will be able to see a change in your body measurements.

Step 10: Things to keep in mind

If you are getting started with Intermittent Fasting or you want to try this diet, then there are a couple of things that you will need to keep in mind. You need to understand that an initial couple of days might be quite hard. Your body will take some time to get accustomed to the new diet and during this time, you need to fight your urge to give in. You need to stick to this diet for at least three weeks before you can see a visible change in your body. It can be difficult to battle your hunger pangs until your body gets used to fasting. So, you need to come up with ways in which you can do so.

Chapter 13
Reasons for Failure

Anyone who practices intermittent fasting as a lifestyle is bound to experience tremendous benefits including better sleep, increased mental clarity, and ability to better manage food cravings. Many attest to the health benefits and general wellbeing after weeks of practicing this lifestyle.

However, these benefits can only be realized if this lifestyle is practiced correctly. Sadly, people make mistakes and end up losing out on some or all these benefits. For instance, some try to do too much within a short time period while others give up too soon.

By avoiding these common mistakes and applying this healthy lifestyle correctly, you will be successful and will realize the benefits of intermittent fasting a lot sooner than you think.

Common Mistakes with Intermittent Fasting

There are plenty of people who get the basics of this lifestyle the first time around. This is all well and good. However, this is not always the case, and some women still get a few things wrong. Here is a look at some of the common mistakes that people often make and how to avoid them.

Choosing the wrong fasting protocol

There are different fasting protocols allowed so finding the right one is crucial. When determining the right kind of protocol, you need to consider your lifestyle. For instance, how busy is your lifestyle? If you have a demanding occupation, then you may want to find the right protocol for you. Therefore, check out the different intermittent fasting protocols and identify the one that best suits your lifestyle.

Not consuming enough fat

Consuming enough amounts of fat with your meals is important. Fat helps prevent the ups and downs of reactive hypoglycemia and sustains your blood sugar. When you do not take enough fat, your insulin goes up, and blood sugar plays up. Then your blood sugar levels drop, and adrenals must push it back up. This is not a desirable situation at all. Fortunately, good quality, healthy fat can help manage this situation. This is fat sourced from coconut oil or avocado.

Unresolved hormonal issues:

If you have high blood sugar levels, thyroid problems, female hormones imbalance, or adrenal glands challenges, then you shouldn't be cutting out those meals just yet. This is because your body is already suffering a physiology problem. If your body is not nourished early morning and early afternoon, then your body may be stressed out. You should first consider getting these issues sorted out first by health practitioner then seek advice about leading an intermittent fasting lifestyle.

Not consuming sufficient calories

Fasting tends to affect the hormones that regulate hunger such that you won't feel as hungry. This way, you are likely to consume very little food. You need to be very careful not to consume too few calories because your body will be deprived of essential nutrition. You should eat at least 1200 calories as a minimum. If you do not do this, then you will feel extremely hungry the following day, and this could affect your ability to perform.

You are scared of feeling hungry

Many people get scared of feeling hungry in the course of the day due to fasting. Yet we all feel hungry at some point during the day even if we consume six meals per day. The problem with this kind of issue is that people often want to eat the minute they feel hungry. The truth is that your body can go without a meal for lengthy periods of time, even 24 hours.

You consume too much junk food

Intermittent fasting is never about what you eat but when you eat. While this is a good mantra to abide by, it sometimes results in problems due to the foods we eat. Most people do not know what to eat. Yet it is possible to consume sumptuous meals that are healthy and good for you. Your focus should be more on animal and plant products, both of which should be unprocessed. While this sounds like a paleo diet, it simply refers to having any meats and fish. Also, eat foods that grow in the garden such as vegetables, fruits, grains, and pulses, and much more. You can consume some processed foods as well. However, try to eat mostly natural foods.

You do not lead an active lifestyle

It is very important to stay busy throughout your fasting period. If you are not busy, then you tend to feel hungry and want to eat anything and everything on site. It is important, especially when starting out, to always keep busy and avoid sitting idle. You can try to schedule something so that you are not around food. Basically, if food is not around, then you will not be tempted. Avoid places with free donuts or where you have friends having meals or snacks.

Abusing stimulants

It is not uncommon for women to take too much coffee. This is wrong because you can end up with a caffeinated euphoria. It is okay to have one or two cups to kick-start your fast day. What you need to avoid is becoming over-reliant on coffee to get through the day. If you must, drink a cup or two and leave it at that. Try not to consume more coffee after your lunch break.

You start off way too ambitious

All too often, people start a diet program or a healthy lifestyle like intermittent fasting with high expectations. It takes most people a long time to get used to hunger and coping with it. You should not be too hard on yourself and do not be too ambitious. Going from regular eating to a single meal per day can come as quite a shock to most people. Go easy on yourself and cut yourself some slack. You should not try to achieve everything all at once but, instead, try to take one step at a time.

You think that more is better

Sometimes people tend to think that fasting for longer means better outcomes and better results. This is not necessarily the case. While intermittent fasting for 16 hours per day is recommended, you should not fast beyond 20 to 24 hours. You will do more harm than good if you increase your fasting hours unnecessarily. In fact, according to a recent study, most fasting benefits begin to dwindle past the 20-hour mark.

Being obsessed with time

Some people are obsessed with time and cannot be flexible. You need to embrace a relaxed lifestyle without undue concern about hours, seconds, and minutes. Basically, an obsessed person stares at the clock and thinks that a single minute past time will ruin their entire fast experience. Many experienced people will eat anytime within their eating window without worrying about the minutes or seconds. If you freed yourself from the 6-meals-a-day program, then you should free yourself from the clock.

Some tend to give up too soon

Intermittent fasting is a lifestyle that requires a certain amount of discipline. It also takes a bit of time to get used to. Health and nutrition experts know that the initial four to five days are the most challenging. You can expect to feel, exhausted, lightheaded, and hungry. The best part is that these feelings will pass quickly and, by the end of the first week, the body will begin to adapt. You will begin to feel more focused, energetic, and your hunger will diminish and eventually disappear. Therefore, rather than giving up too soon, assess your situation after the first week and see if you can make any adjustments.

Working out excessively

If you are physically unfit and are just starting out with intermittent fasting, then be very careful not to do anything excessively, especially exercising. The best approach to exercising is to ease yourself into a routine. In fact, both fasting and exercising require a gradual approach. It would be disastrous as a beginner to join a 5-day intense workout program. Your body is already trying to adjust to limited food intake, so an intense workout can lead to fatigue and possibly hospitalization. A little bit of physical strain now and then is good for the body but too much all at once can be a problem.

Chapter 14
Intermittent Fasting Myths

Like most popular elements of the world, intermittent fasting has its share of myths that need to be broken to clearly and unambiguously understand the way it operates. So, let's go and bust some myths.

Intermittent fasting will lead us into starvation mode —People are led to believe that intermittent fasting will put our bodies into a starvation mode because our brain gets the signal that it is 'famine time' lowering its rate of metabolism. This is nothing but a myth. Studies have shown that our bodies do not lower their metabolic rates unless and until you have not given it nourishment for at least three entire days.

Since our cavemen days, the human body has been developed to withstand days of famine. How can a few hours of not eating anything put your body on the defensive? Starvation mode starts only when the body has completely used up all its fat reserves. Only at this stage will our body break down muscle. Your body will not touch your muscles if you skipped a meal or two, and definitely not if you have only skipped breakfast!

Intermittent fasting compels your body to use up stored fat while keeping your lean mass intact. If you have excessive fat in your body, then intermittent fasting can work wonders because it will reach out for these reserves almost immediately after it has completely utilized the energy from your last meal.

With Intermittent fasting, you have the freedom to eat anything you want during the eating window – Unfortunately, this myth is also the biggest pitfall for novices to fall into as they struggle to make intermittent fasting work. Yes, you have fasted for a certain period. But that does not give you the freedom to eat whatever you want once the fasting period is over.

Losing weight from intermittent fasting is also based on a caloric deficit. If you exceed your daily calorie needs, you will never lose weight. The number of calories that your body continuously burns throughout the day to maintain your current body weight is what is referred to as daily calorific needs.

Your daily calorie intake is dependent on a whole lot of factors including your age, gender, body fat, weight, height, physical activity levels, profession, and more. If you consume more calories than your body burns during your eating window, then you will gain weight irrespective of how long you fasted for before it.

You must be watchful of how many calories you are consuming to ensure you stay within the required range. Additionally, your meals must include plenty of fresh fruits and vegetables to meet your body's fiber needs. Excessively fatty foods, processed foods, food with preservatives should be avoided. Nutritious, wholesome, and fresh foods are your best bet.

Intermittent fasting will make you feel hungry always – A great worry that people have about intermittent fasting is that they will have to stay hungry for 16, 18, or even 20 hours. In the minds of novices, this means being hungry almost every minute of the day! This is a total myth.

Initially, intermitting fasting is going to make you uncomfortable because your body has got accustomed to receiving food at frequent intervals and hasn't got an opportunity to reach out to the stored fat reserves. Your body and mind are going to take a little bit of time getting used to the paradigm shift in energy consumption.

But, once your body understands that the energy reserves are right there for it to take (and, plenty of it, too), it will cease to create unpleasant and uncomfortable sensations for you. Your body will automatically shift its metabolic mechanism to adapt to your new eating methods. Hunger pangs will disappear after the initial adjustment.

Starting slowly is a great way to manage hunger pangs. Start with the 12-hour fasting period, then move to the 14 hours, and then to the 16 hours. This way, your body will not unduly send out hunger pangs signals. Always listen to your body and move forward gradually for maximum effect. The 18-hour period should typically be your aim. However, the 16:8 method can work wonders too.

Intermittent fasting is a 'magical' trick – Nothing can be farther from the truth. Yes, it might seem like magic considering the quick and effective results it can produce. But multiple scientific studies have proven the efficacy of intermittent fasting in bringing about the desired outcomes using basic human metabolism.

Moreover, you already know that fasting is not some new-age weight-loss dieting cult. It has been around for thousands of years as a natural healing and cleansing process. The recent scientific studies only support what our ancestors already knew and followed on a day-to-day basis.

The basic science behind intermittent fasting is simple. If you spend more calories than you consume, your body will be in caloric deficit. And, it will use up fat reserves for the differential energy resulting in fat/weight loss. If the value of one pound of fat is 3500 calories, then reducing 500 calories from your base metabolic rate will result in a loss of one pound of weight every week.

Intermittent fasting is just another crash/fad diet – One of the first things you learned about intermittent fasting is that it is not a diet. It is only a pattern of eating. Theoretically, if you consume fewer calories than what you spend, your meal can be pizza and beer, too. However, in practice, this approach will not work because eating only pizza and beer will never help you get all the essential nutrients your body needs for healthy living.

Intermittent fasting is, therefore, only a guide and tells you clearly WHEN you should NOT eat. It is not a fad or crash diet that promises you miracles if you stay away from or eat certain types of food.

Chapter 15
Intermittent Fasting as A Lifestyle

If you want to stick to intermittent fasting for life, then you must not view it as a diet but as a lifestyle. This will require you to reevaluate your eating choices, even before beginning the fast, so that when you begin, you are sure that you won't be going back. For example, if you use regular vegetable oil, then it is time to replace it with healthy oils such as coconut oil and olive oil. If you tend to eat processed carbs, then it is time to replace them with healthy whole, unprocessed carbs- e.g., zucchini noodles in place of pasta.

The idea here is to embrace the diet and the fact that your body will be a full-on fat burning means that new carbs won't be required for body fuel. It will take a few weeks for this to happen, but once it does, cravings for unhealthy carbs will be out of the picture and incorporating this diet into your life will be as easy as ABC.

If you are going to live the ultimate intermittent fasting lifestyle then:

The best way to include Intermittent Fasting into your lifestyle is by delaying your breakfast slowly by slowly; delay by an hour then another hour the next day and so on. Take an hour to shower, an hour to do your chores, an hour to get to work. Just take an hour from any activity that you engage in the morning that you see the best fit until you get to a time that you can live with.

Do not use fasting as an excuse to eat junk; calories are different. 100 calories of broccoli are not the same as 100 calories of a snicker bar. When you find yourself cheating then get real with yourself. Keep the carbs for before workouts and fill yourself up with meats and veggies.

Stick to the method that you are most comfortable with, as discussed; there are a number of ways to do intermittent fasting. Play around with all of them and get what suits you best. Make sure you try out all methods; you might be surprised which will be easiest to follow. In order to make something part of your lifestyle, you need to be fully comfortable with it. Intermittent fasting is no different.

Chapter 16
Lessons Acquired from
Intermittent Fasting

People who have tried this method of fasting have reported getting stronger and leaner, without giving up their favorite foods and feeling cranky. They have also experienced certain life lessons while undergoing fasting, some of which are listed below. Look at them as an inspirational guide to get you started on your own journey.

Your mind is your biggest barrier.

If you look at it objectively, this diet is simple to implement. Depending on the kind of fasting you do, you skip certain meals and make up for them at other times. The biggest hurdle here is telling your mind to accept the changes. People think that if they don't eat at the designated time, they might faint or fall sick. They think that they need to eat every two or three hours, and not skip breakfast at all or have a light dinner. Once you get started on this fasting, you will realize how easy and simple it is, and how much healthier you feel from the inside. It usually helps most people to ease into it slowly. It goes against much of what you have likely been taught and therefore you think you know about your body and your health. You will change your mind about that once you see the effects of periodic fasting in action, and over time your fears and apprehensions will be proven to be unfounded. You'll find yourself healthier and more energetic than ever. The hardest part is taking that leap and starting.

It is easy to lose weight and keep it that way.

When the number of calories you ingest is less than the number of calories you burn, you lose weight. It's as simple as that. Intermittent fasting allows one to lose weight without losing muscle mass. It is a great option for people who are looking to lose weight because the weight loss happens without any change in the diet or foods. The only thing which changes is the time when you eat your food. People lose weight with this method because when they eliminate meals from their time plan and they don't binge eat at the next feeding.

It is possible to build muscle while fasting.

People who have tried intermittent fasting have reported gaining lean body mass and cutting body fat by as much as five percent. This happens due to the body's tendency to lose weight during the fasting period. Your body begins to utilize the fat stores you have built up for energy when it does not have readily accessible energy sources from food. But you do not go so long without that your muscle supply becomes fodder for energy. At the end of the day, your caloric intake is the same. Whether you ingest two thousand calories during a 16 hours or 24-hour span or 8-hour span does not matter. You just need to eat enough to build muscle.

It results in more productivity, at least for some people.

Some people have stated that they experience a lot of mental clarity during their fasting periods. Contrary to popular belief, fasting does not drain the body and mind of energy. Letting go of your focus on and preoccupation with food can enable you to think about and apply your creativity to other interests and activities. No longer do you have to consider what you will make for dinner that night and if you have the time. Instead, the day is truly yours, with no need to shop, cook, wash dishes, or even waste your precious time eating. You can focus your mind solely on your interests and desires, as opposed to distracting yourself with something you once thought was a necessity.

Cycling your foods might be the way to go.

Intermittent fasting will work much better when you start cycling your foods and calorie combinations. For instance, eat a bit more when you are going to work out and a bit less when you are on a rest period. This means you will have a calorie surplus on the days you train, and a deficit on the days you rest. By doing this, you build muscle on the days you work out, and you burn body fat while you rest. You need to ensure you have the calories and nutrients to use on the days you are working hard in order to gain and keep lean muscle mass. When you want to take it easy and relax, it should be simple enough just not to eat while you do it. After all, it's nothing more than a mental exercise. You don't physically require the food as much when you are not as active. Your body will just naturally go through your fat stores, and you will be closer than ever to achieving your fitness goals and shedding that excess body fat. Keep cycling your carbs and protein with the days you train and rest. This will lead you to become leaner, with elevated muscle mass and low body fat levels

Chapter 17
Intermittent Fasting FAQ

Can I drink coffee while I am fasting?

Coffee is a beverage that millions of people enjoy each day. This is why many people are concerned that they might have to give up their cup of coffee that they enjoy so much each morning if they are going to start following an intermittent fasting plan. The majority of these plans will tell you to sustain from eating until later in the afternoon and to skip on breakfast for a boost in benefits.

Fortunately, there is no need to worry if you are planning to implement intermittent fasting into your diet – and would still like to have a cup or two of coffee in the morning. There is, however, one factor that you do need to note here. If you want to have a cup of coffee after waking up and your intermittent fasting plan demands that you continue with your fasting window in the morning, then it means no sugar and no milk for you. While some people have noted that it is okay to add one splash of milk to your coffee while fasting, this is usually not recommended if you are serious about losing weight while you are following an intermittent fasting plan.

Coffee can be a great addition to your diet plan and be a good boost for getting through that last period of fasting. When you opt for a cup of coffee in the morning, you will get an energy boost – and since the caffeine in coffee may provide you with benefits for as long as six hours, you can easily glide on these effects until the time comes to break your fasting period.

Coffee has also been shown to speed up metabolism, which is great for anyone looking to lose weight. You'll end up burning even more fat.

Additionally, coffee will help to keep your mind sharp during the morning and avoid those dreadful times when brain fog hits you because you are running on empty.

There is another benefit that should be noted in terms of having a cup of coffee for breakfast, instead of indulging in a big breakfast. This particular benefit comes in handy for those who are looking to work out while they are still fasting – many people prefer a morning workout, after all. Some people follow an intermittent fasting plan that finds they do not have the same level of energy while working out compared to eating a good breakfast before they go out and hit the gym. When you drink some coffee, you'll get a boost in both physical performances, and cognitive function – both are crucial for a good workout in the gym.

Should I break my fast with a big or small meal?

Another popular question that people tend to ask when it comes to intermittent fasting is how exactly they should break their fast. The opinions in regard to breaking a fasting window while following an intermittent fasting program is mixed. Some suggest that you break the fast with a big meal that is packed with calories to load your body with protein and other essential nutrients, while others suggest that you start out simple and small, and then gradually work up to that big meal.

There really isn't a single perfect answer to this question, but it should be considered that when breaking a fast, the body is still in a fat burning mode. When you hit your body with too many calories at once, you can switch off this mode and experience less of the benefits that you are expecting from your intermittent fasting plan.

Thus, it is generally not considered a good idea to break your fast with a meal that is considered loaded in calories. I personally find that it is much more convenient to start things out slowly. Perhaps break that fasting period with a green salad, or perhaps some Greek yogurt. Many options can help to satisfy the hunger you have built up during the fast, offer you a series of healthy and essential nutrients, but without causing your metabolism to shut down.

After the fast has been broken and you have had your first meal, plan for a second and a third meal as well. Be sure that these meals will also be nutritious and healthy. I enjoy a big meal that makes up most of the calories I should consume daily by the end of the day. Some might prefer this "big meal" to happen in between their first and third meal – this way, they can start their eating cycle and end the cycle with something small. This would also help to reduce the number of calories you should consume just before you go to bed.

A good idea would also be to experiment with different options. Try to make the second meal of the eating period your big meal of the day. See how your body reacts. You might also try the first and the final meal of the day – make these your big meals. Really observe how you feel with each of these options. You'll eventually start to notice that your body reacts better to one of these options – or perhaps spreading out your calories equally. When you find the right option, continue with it.

How do I cope with my hunger during the fasting window?

When you are starting out with intermittent fasting for the first time and you are used to eating three or more meals a day, along with some snacking in-between, then there really is no doubt that for the initial period of intermittent fasting, you will experience hunger and some cravings. This is something that most people struggle with – and it is an issue that often causes people to give up on intermittent fasting and either return to their usual way of eating or turn to another type of diet to help them possibly lose the excess weight that is causing them concern.

The key to success in terms of coping with hunger when starting with an intermittent fasting program really is patience. You will need to have patience when it comes to feeling the effects of this diet come into play. It will take some time, but when you push through these hunger strikes, you will start to notice the cravings become fewer and fewer as the days go by. Instead of experiencing cravings for candy and other unhealthy foods, you will start to experience hunger – this is a good thing, so do not think of the hunger as a bad thing that is striking you at the most unpleasant times.

Since you are not craving unhealthy foods, you will be less likely to start searching for donuts and candy bars to snack on. You will find that it is easier to push through until you reach the time where you can have your first meal.

If you do feel that you are unable to cope anymore and those last few hours simply seem too far away, then have sparkling water. This will help to make your stomach feel full for a little while – in turn, you will find that it becomes much easier to last for an hour or two more in order to reach the time when you can finally break your fast.

How will I train if I am running empty on food?

While coping with hunger is one thing that people struggle with when they are following an intermittent fasting plan, another issue that some also find is that they are not sure how they will continue with their training regime once they start to follow this type of program. The obvious idea behind intermittent fasting is that you would find yourself running low on food just in the nick of time when you decide to hit the gym – this means you do not have an adequate source of fuel to give you that energy you need to push through the entire session.

Some people actually find that they can train more efficiently when their stomach is not full. There are also many who have claimed training during a fasting period is more beneficial – and that it is sometimes even easier.

If you do feel that you are unable to get through that upcoming training session because you feel "empty" and out of energy, then perhaps consider opting for a cup of coffee – no milk or sugar, however. The coffee will give you the boost you need to get through the entire session and may even give you some energy afterward to last until the time at which you can break the fast.

Keep in mind that when training on an empty stomach, your body will not have food to turn to to generate energy. In turn, this also means that your body will start to turn to the fat storages within your body in order to generate the energy that you need to continue running on that treadmill or to continue pushing those weights. This, in turn, also means fat is burnt faster and much more effectively.

Is it okay to cheat now-and-then?

When it comes to fasting for weight loss, people are usually inclined to follow a specific meal plan and diet that will give them guidance on what they can eat during the periods that they can consume calories. In most cases, diets will be somewhat restricted – they will usually include healthy foods that are relatively low in carbohydrates while being high in protein and other essential nutrients.

The healthy meals will surely make you feel great, but there is no shame in wanting to have a "cheat" snack or even a cheat meal now-and-then. The big question now is whether it is okay for you to have a cheat day, or even just a cheat snack or treat.

Having a "cheat" day will not do you a lot of harm in terms of your weight loss results – the important part here is to ensure that this does not happen every day. Try to limit yourself to a cheat once a week at most. Perhaps grab a bar of chocolate from your local supermarket or, if you really want to go bigger, get your family to agree to dinner at a local restaurant.

When you do have a cheat day or meal, it is important that you take the calories consumed while 'cheating' into account. This number of calories you will have to make up for the next day – this way, you'll continue to experience the benefits of the diet.

Consider the number of calories you went over your daily limit today – perhaps that bar of chocolate added another 150 calories to your day.

Conclusion

Thank you again for downloading this book! I hope it provided you with the understanding of the wide variety of options you have when it comes to intermittent fasting and how you can best mix and match to find the perfect solution for you. Deciding to alter your primary eating patterns is a major one, and it is important that you take the full weight of the decision into account before acting.

If you have what it takes to take full advantage of the benefits that intermittent fasting has to offer, then the next step is to stop reading and to start fasting. Choose the type of intermittent fasting that seems the best fit for you and give it a try.

Don't be discouraged if you don't receive immediate results. Try to find the one that's right for you. Above all, don't rush, and remember, intermittent fasting is a marathon not a sprint, slow and steady will win the race.

Lastly, if you found this book useful in any way, a review on Amazon is always appreciated!

Bonus Material: Earning – An Introduction To Earning With The Double Your Income Sequence

SECTION 1: THE SECRET OF FORMING MONEY HABITS (AND HOW TO ENFORCE THEM)

You are a collection of your favorite habits.

And, you have a niche set of habits that contribute to the money you can earn and keep, during your average month. Understanding the science behind these habits will help you positively influence the energy you spend on making more money.

A habit is a practice that you have used so often, that it has become an internalized, autonomic blueprint – a kind of default program for how to execute a specific action.[1]

Habits become damaging when they stop being beneficial, and instead, become uncontrollable, unintentional and contrary to your personal goals. Most individuals carry with them the burden of many bad habits, which inadvertently keeps them from forging ahead and achieving their income goals.

According to Charles Duhigg, the reason why we struggle with habits is that they are as unique as we are. There is no quick-fix formula.

---

[1] Habit, Wikipedia, https://en.wikipedia.org/wiki/Habit

14

In order to effectively change your habits, you need enlightenment on a better process, and, on your stuck behavior. Then you can change your *cue-routine-reward* cycle.[2]

Cue: a trigger that puts your brain in automatic mode and chooses your habit

Routine: A physical, mental or emotional set of actions

Reward: What you gain from executing the habit

With fresh ideas and an understanding of how to break bad habit loops, you will adopt powerful new habits that will help you double your income every, single, month.

SECTION 2: HOW TO CREATE NEW MONEY HABITS

New habits are how you will double your income.

This means you need to:

---

[2] Duhigg, Charles, How Habits Work, https://charlesduhigg.com/how-habits-work/

#1: Identify and break bad habits, to free up room for fresh practices

#2: Identity and consciously adopt new habits, until they become automatic

This guide is not about the first step. If you want to learn how to break bad habits, I suggest reading Charles Duhigg's classic, "The Power of Habit."

What you do need to realize, is that a number of your existing habits need to change, to make room for the ones outlined in this guide. You must become consciously aware of your *cue-routine-reward cycle*, and interrupt it to stay on track.

You can do this effectively by replacing your existing rewards, with your new goal to double your income. To create a new habit, follow this simple process.

> **Identify the bad habit that must be replaced**

>> Waking up at 7 am to be at work at 8 am

> **Identify the harm it's causing**

>> Rushing and feeling harassed and irritated when you get to work

> **Understand and replace the reward from your bad habit**

Instead of instant gratification from sleeping late, your mood will be elevated, and your energy levels will be high at work

> **Implement the new habit, motivated by a stronger overall reward**

Practice waking up at 5 am, arriving at work at 7:30 and easing into your day, to stimulate the positive mindset required for success

According to modern studies, it takes roughly 66 days before a new behavior becomes automatic.[3]

SECTION 3: THE 14 HABITS THAT WILL DOUBLE YOUR INCOME

Here are the habits you need.

Habit 1: SLEEP (You're Not Doing It Right)

Bill Gates, the co-founder of Microsoft, sleeps for 7 hours every night and reads for 1 hour before bedtime.

With over a third of Americans not getting enough regular sleep, most people vastly underestimate the importance of quality shuteye in their lives.

Over or under-sleeping exposes you to increased risk for chronic conditions, mental distress, stroke and heart disease.[4] According to a 2018 Poll by The National Sleep Foundation, excellent sleepers feel more effective at getting things done the next day.[5]

---

[3] Lally, Phillippa, How are Habits Formed: Modelling Habit Formation in the Real World, https://onlinelibrary.wiley.com/doi/abs/10.1002/ejsp.674

[4] 1 in 3 Adults Don't Get Enough Sleep, https://www.cdc.gov/media/releases/2016/p0215-enough-sleep.html

[5] National Sleep Foundation's 2018 Sleep in America Poll Shows Americans Failing to Prioritize Sleep, https://sleepfoundation.org/media-center/press-release/2018-sleep-in-america-poll-shows

The first habit you need to adopt is simple – get high quality, regular sleep.

Set a time every evening to go to sleep and stick to it. You should be in bed an hour before, your phone off and all screens far away from you. Read for an hour. Then, go to sleep for 7.

Wake up promptly, 7 hours later. Not a minute more.

Sticking to this new habit promises you stronger immunity, the improved concentration at work and greater emotional stability overall. Consistency will ensure that your circadian rhythms function well, and you never have trouble with restless sleep or with falling asleep.[6]

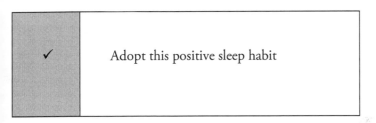

✓   Adopt this positive sleep habit

Habit 2: EXERCISE (It's Not Enough, or It's Too Much)

Ex-President Barack Obama works out for 45 minutes a day, six days a week. Thirty minutes or more of aerobic exercise is done daily by 76% of all successful people.[7]

Aerobic exercise is the one consistent habit that will give you the energy

---

[6] Mahabir, Nicole, How and Why Waking Up at the Same Time Every Day Can Improve Your Health, https://www.cbc.ca/life/wellness/how-and-why-waking-up-at-the-same-time-everyday-can-improve-your-health-1.4357391

[7] Cohen Jennifer, Exercise is One Thing Most Successful People Do Everyday, https://www.entrepreneur.com/article/276760

you need to succeed. You should run, walk, jog, bike or take a class at the gym. Cardio gets your blood pumping, which is ideal for your brain and boosts your intelligence.[8]

The second habit you need to adopt – find and practice an aerobic exercise, daily.

Now, you need to pick 45 minutes to an hour, every day to get your cardio in. It makes no difference whether you do this in the morning, or late in the evening – as long as it is done every single day.

Consistency is how you will reap these many benefits.

Try to pick something that fits into your life, schedule and likes. You don't have to spend money, you simply have to get active. This means finding an exercise you will enjoy. Some people like boxing classes, others prefer to take a walk around the neighborhood.

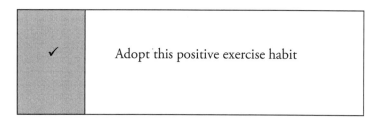

| ✓ | Adopt this positive exercise habit |

Habit 3: SOCIAL ENERGY (Here's One to Protect)

Oprah Winfrey, talk-show host, and owner of Harpo Studios meditates for 20 minutes every morning, shortly after waking up.

---

[8] Regular Exercise Releases Brain Chemicals Key for Memory, Concentration, and Mental Sharpness, From the May 2013 Harvard Men's Health Watch, https://www.health.harvard.edu/press_releases/regular-exercise-releases-brain-chemicals-key-for-memory-concentration-and-mental-sharpness

Meditation makes you more in-tune with yourself, how you feel, and how the world around you feels. It's great for focus, increased energy, decreased stress and lifts brain fog.[9]

The people around you have an impact on your energy levels. Successful people surround themselves with positive, go-getters – while the average person is drained by one or more toxic, or negative people in their lives. Social energy must be protected.

The third habit is – to meditate daily on how to optimize your social energy.

According to a Cigna Study, loneliness is at epidemic levels in America.[10] But this is never a good reason to allow anyone a place in your life.

Take a look at your connections and consider if they add, or take energy away from you as you meditate for 20 minutes every morning.

Extroverted, or introverted, you need the right kind of connections in your daily life. If you have energy vampires in your sphere, you must get rid of them to be at your best.

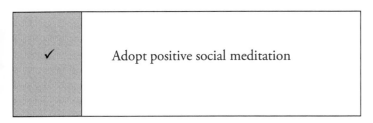

| ✓ | Adopt positive social meditation |

---

[9] Sun, Carolyn, I Tried This Oprah Meditation Hack Every Day for Two Weeks. Here Are My 5 Takeaways, https://www.entrepreneur.com/article/310039

[10] New Cigna Study Reveals Loneliness at Epidemic Levels in America, https://www.prnewswire.com/news-releases/new-cigna-study-reveals-loneliness-at-epidemic-levels-in-america-300639747.html

Habit 4: SELF-INVESTMENT (Knowing and Doing)

Albert Einstein believed in constant self-investment through learning, research and application of that newfound knowledge.

The day you stop learning, is the day you stop growing. And personal growth is what takes you towards income acceleration and success. Einstein knew that constant reading was critical to learning, but so was the application of the knowledge learned while reading.

He famously said that too much reading renders the brain lazy. To grow in his field, Einstein continued to study formally until he was 26, then pursued self-study. He was not, as many believe, a naturally talented genius savant – he studied, read and practiced knowledge.[11]

The fourth habit is – invest in your field of knowledge through reading and practice.

If you want to excel like Einstein, shift from consuming entertainment to consuming knowledge. This is easily done by dedicating an hour or more to reading and applying your newly discovered knowledge. Practice what you learn, to see the real difference.[12]

Carve an hour of your day, in the morning or evening to read a book and then realize its lessons. This can be split into 30 minutes of reading, 30 minutes of creating.

---

[11] Shead, Mark, Are You Reading Too Much?, http://www.productivity501.com/are-you-reading-too-much/8874/

[12] How Much Did Albert Einstein Study?, https://www.forbes.com/sites/quora/2017/12/28/how-much-did-albert-einstein-study/#1595adeb28bc

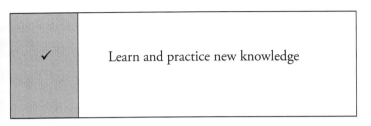

✓	Learn and practice new knowledge

Habit 5: DELEGATION (Focus on The Big Picture)

Richard Branson, Founder of Virgin and hundreds of other companies, is famous for his practice of 'letting go, to grow.' He delegates to focus on the big picture.[13]

Delegation is a habit that most people fail to practice. Instead, they try to do everything themselves and end up burned out, exhausted and depleted.

When you actively practice delegation, you become a talented multitasker, able to orchestrate and design your own career. It is at this point your income will inflate.

The fifth habit is – to practice delegation often and keep your eyes on the big picture.

Your career, or income goals, maybe the big picture for now. Knowing where you want to end up gives you clarity of purpose, and will help you assign what is not important to those around you. This must be done in all aspects of your life that consume your time.

---

[13] Richard Branson: Why Delegation is Crucial for Success,
https://www.virgin.com/entrepreneur/richard-branson-why-delegation-crucial-success

This habit will kick in when someone makes demands on your time. Ask yourself if it contributes to your big picture. If it does not, find a creative way of delegating it to another human being. Make this a habit, and soon you will be surrounded by competent people.[14]

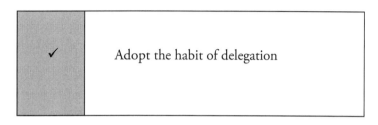

✓   Adopt the habit of delegation

Habit 6: MENTORING (Learning and Teaching)

Marie Forleo is a life coach, philanthropist and entrepreneur, who believes in the power of mentoring and being mentored, to become hugely successful.[15]

In fact, she uses connections to grow her business at every level. With storytelling and the ability to build a community around her lifestyle brand, she was named Oprah's *"thought leader for the next generation."*

Your ability to surround yourself with the right people will be the single most useful habit you can adopt. Most people never actively practice the art of conscious mentoring.

The sixth habit is – to practice attracting network connections that will help you excel!

---

[14] Coleman, Alison, Delegate Like Branson: Hire People Who are More Talented Than You, https://www.forbes.com/sites/alisoncoleman/2015/01/25/delegate-like-branson-hire-people-who-are-more-talented-than-you/#4ce10d27cb3d

[15] Brouwer, Allen, Lavery, Cathryn, Why Marie Forleo Says This One Marketing Trick Is So Important, https://www.entrepreneur.com/article/305586

Who do you know that could teach you something important? Have you ever met someone who you wanted to learn from? Teaching and learning is fundamental to networking, and the basis for all positive relationships, in a corporate environment.[16]

Every day, you should consciously invest more energy in stimulating and improving mentor relationships that will help you grow and succeed as a person in your field. Be ruthlessly selective about your friends and who you spend the most time with.

Allow others to mentor you, and be mentored by you, in a working environment.

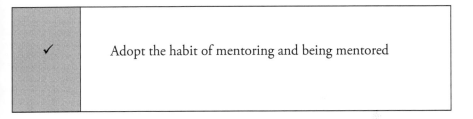

✔ Adopt the habit of mentoring and being mentored

Habit 7: YOUR 96 MINUTES (This is Your Most Valuable Time)

Stephen King is known for his work ethic and ability to produce six good pages of writing every day consistently. He does this by following the same productivity routine daily. [17]

---

[16] Forleo, Marie, Networking For Introverts W/Susan Cain, https://www.marieforleo.com/2013/11/susan-cain-introverts-networking/

[17] Cotterill, Thomas, Stephen Kings Work Habits, https://thomascotterill.wordpress.com/2012/09/13/stephen-kings-work-habits/

You need to have the discipline and consistency required, to do something for your direct productivity benefit, for 96 minutes a day. Why 96 minutes?

Science says that everyone has 96 highly productive minutes every day, a time window when you have the most energy and are at your best. If you harness this power and use it for your ultimate goal of earning more money, it shifts from possible, to probable.[18]

The seventh habit is – Spend 96 minutes a day working on your main career goal.

Discover when your 96 minutes kicks in. It might be just after waking up. It might be late at night when everyone else is sleeping. Find your window and use it.

Spend those 96 minutes focused exclusively on your main career goal. If that is to get a promotion, this is when you will plan and execute a strategy. If it is to launch a website, this is when you will put in the work.

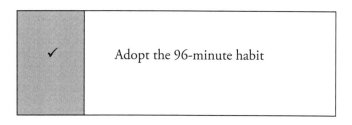

✔	Adopt the 96-minute habit

---

[18] The Rule of 96 Minutes to Productivity, http://sapience.net/blog/the-rule-of-96-minutes-to-productivity/

Habit 8: INNOVATION (Get to The Core of Things)

Elon Musk, the founder of PayPal, SpaceX and Tesla, is a known innovator and practices the Richard Feynman technique mixed with first principles, to stay creative. [19]

The underlying concept of this technique is to not try and remember, but to understand – because when you do, you automatically remember. It's a way to entertain new ideas and be creative in a way that promotes productivity.

Knowledge to Elon, is about understanding the fundamental principles of a thing, to know the trunk and branches before diving headlong into the details, or the leaves of an idea.

The eighth habit is – when learning something new, to understand its core first.

Applying this to your career will make you a forward-thinking innovator. For example, if you are a psychologist, you would benefit from learning more about neuroscience, because it is at the core of your field. Competency is all about strong, unshakable fundamentals.[20]

Spend 30 minutes every day learning something that reinforces how you innovate in your chosen field. Soon you will be questioning, brainstorming and seeing patterns that may amount to improvements you can implement.

---

[19] The Feynman Technique: The Best Way to Learn Anything, https://fs.blog/2012/04/learn-anything-faster-with-the-feynman-technique/

[20] Stillman, Jessica, 3 Smart Strategies Genuises Like Albert Einstein and Elon Musk Use to Learn Anything Faster, http://www.businessinsider.com/3-strategies-geniuses-like-elon-musk-use-to-learn-anything-faster-2017-10?IR=T

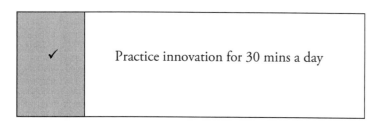

| ✓ | Practice innovation for 30 mins a day |

Habit 9: THE WIN-WIN (Mutually Beneficial Relationships)

Stephen Covey, author of the smash hit "The 7 Habits of Highly Effective People" advocated the importance of win-win relationships.

According to Covey, most people approach life with a scarcity mindset, as opposed to an abundance mindset. Because of this, social interactions become unbalanced.[21]

There are several types of human interaction, win-lose, lose-lose, lose-win – but none are as powerful or effective as the win-win. When you practice win-win interactions, your engagements are mutually beneficial, and people will enjoy working with you.

The ninth habit is – to practice win-win human interactions in your daily life.

When you do, you will find that people flock to you, because they see the benefits of doing business with you. When everyone benefits, you can succeed together.

This habit will cue when someone asks you for something. This should be your trigger to think about how you can make the interaction a win-

---

[21] Hussain, Anum, 7 Habits of Highly Effective People [Book Summary], https://blog.hubspot.com/sales/habits-of-highly-effective-people-summary

win scenario. Covey says, to take consideration and courage into account, and to be creative in your problem-solving.

As you create win-win results, your influence will grow in your field. Remember that there is enough success around for everyone, and you can create it for them!

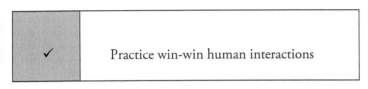

✓   Practice win-win human interactions

Habit 10: SPEAK UP (Know and Communicate Your Value)

Tyra Banks, ex-supermodel, TV producer and personality, based her career success on the ability to speak up, negotiate and get what she desires most.

She made a habit of speaking clearly, frankly and openly about her value with the people around her. Too often, we get stuck in the habit of remaining passive, and silent about our worth. Promotions and opportunities will pass you by because you failed to speak up.

The tenth habit is – to speak up when necessary about your value as an employee.

Tyra explains, that it is a shift from an 'I need' to an 'I deserve' mindset. Instead of explaining to your employer why you need a raise, you should explain why you deserve one. This is easily done by focusing on your value – or how you positively contribute to the company.[22]

This is another habit that will cue when you identify opportunities or feel

---

[22] Atalla, Jen, Tyra Banks on How to Ask for a Raise,
http://www.businessinsider.com/tyra-banks-how-to-ask-for-a-raise-2018-4?IR=T

that you deserve a promotion at your job. In meetings, be open about your contributions to the success of projects or initiatives. Speak up about how you, as a person, make things better.

Getting into the habit of communicating your worth to people around you, positions you for rapid advancement. If you cannot see and communicate your value, the higher-ups will not see it either. Be persistent. Have a clear voice. And do not get lost in the crowd.

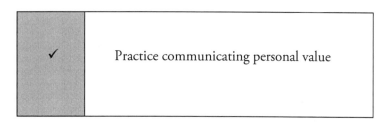

✓   Practice communicating personal value

Habit 11: PAY YOURSELF FIRST (This is Ground-breaking Advice)

George Clason was the author who wrote the classic 'The Richest Man in Babylon' and taught people to pay themselves first, in order to gain real wealth.[23]

Imagine if, since you had started working at age 21, you had put away 10% of every paycheck. This is what it means to pay yourself first. Money saved and kept earns compound interest and grows exponentially over long periods of time.

People that want to be wealthy use this strategy to move from employed

---

[23] Canfield, Jack, The Key to Wealth: Pay Yourself First,
http://jackcanfield.com/blog/the-key-to-wealth-pay-yourself-first/

earning to investing. Investing money is how you break out of your income bracket altogether.

The eleventh habit is – to put 10% of every paycheck aside to grow your wealth.

It might seem like very little at first, but 5 years of putting away just $100.00, frees up $6000.00 for investment. It gives you options to supplement your salary as you age.

To start the habit, every time you are paid – immediately take 10% of that total amount and put it in a separate account. You cannot touch this money. It is there simply to exist and earn you money from long-term growth.

The pay yourself first habit will help you clear away your debt, and get you investing at a young age. Get into this habit early, and you will benefit from time itself.

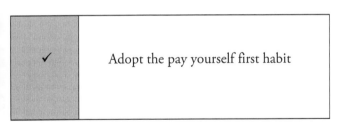

✓   Adopt the pay yourself first habit

Habit 12: SIDE HUSTLE (Spend Your Time for Returns)

Rob Kalin never meant Etsy.com to be such a smash success. Initially, it was simply his side hustle, born from a desire to make wood-encased computers. [24]

Rob Kalin is a furniture designer who started Etsy as a place to sell his wares. It was a side hustle, an increasingly common play among Millennials. Some 61% of Millennials work on their side hustles once a week or more.[25]

This is usually a job that earns them money beyond their 9-5, or a personal project with income potential that they are developing. What is your side hustle?

The twelfth habit is – work on your side hustle twice a week.

On Mondays and Thursdays, or Tuesdays and Fridays you should dedicate a couple of hours to your side hustle. This is a second business, born from your creative or analytical talents that may become a solid earner for you down the line.

Scheduling in time to develop your secondary projects is important for personal growth, and increasing your income. Many Millennials discover that once their side businesses reach a certain level, they can either sell them or commit fulltime to their passions.

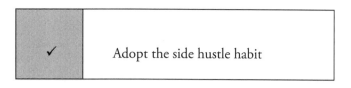

✓   Adopt the side hustle habit

---

[24] Green, Penelope, Scratching an Itch,
https://www.nytimes.com/2016/05/05/style/etsy-rob-kalin.html

[25] Sophy, Joshua, More Than 1 in 4 Millennials Work a Side Hustle,
https://smallbiztrends.com/2017/07/millennial-side-hustle-statistics.html

Habit 13: SUNDAY REVIEW (3 Hours to Financial Freedom!)

Suze Orman, a personal finance expert and personality, is known for teaching people to pick just one thing about their finances to work on, at a time. [26]

She called it the 'one and done' method, and it simplifies the huge challenge of getting hold of your financial situation. Many people find their finances overwhelming, and so never take proactive steps towards understanding and controlling them.

The thirteenth habit is – to spend 3 hours every Sunday focusing on one financial problem.

You might need to save, or clear debt, or better understand your expenses and how to curb them. Whatever you need, you will tackle it during a designated time, every Sunday.

When you practice the habit of reviewing your finances regularly, to better understand and control them, you will change your life.

Make sure that you pick only one simple thing at a time so that you can properly digest and institute changes as necessary. Spend the time learning and streamlining for your ultimate benefit, as a responsible financial planner.

---

[26] Financial Resolutions for 2017? Just Do This One Thing,
https://www.suzeorman.com/blog/financial-resolutions-for-2017-just-do-this-one-thing

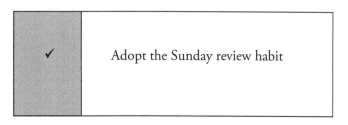

| ✓ | Adopt the Sunday review habit |

Habit 14: MINIMALISM (Know How to Spend)

Steve Jobs, Founder of Apple, was a noted minimalist and wore the same black turtleneck every day for many, many years.

Popularized by Silicon Valley, minimalism reduces decision-fatigue, a common problem in today's overcrowded, ultra-informed society. With so much information and choice out there, it is no wonder you struggle to make good decisions for yourself.[27]

The theory goes that you can only make so many strong decisions in a day. The minimalist habit, allows you to dedicate those decisions to things that matter, like spending for value.

The fourteenth habit is – to spend with minimalism in mind.

Consumer culture is not for the truly rich. Instead, these individuals spend more money on a single item of quality, than repeated spending on numerous low-quality items.

Get into the habit of spending money on quality items, instead of cheaper items that will wear and degrade. This will free up your time as you make fewer wardrobe decisions. Instead of spending your creative energy there, you will spend it at work, where it matters most.

---

[27] Steve Jobs and Minimalism, http://www.applegazette.com/ipod/steve-jobs-and-minimalism/

Less items of higher quality will simplify and improve your life.

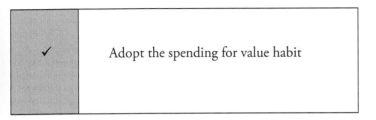

| ✓ | Adopt the spending for value habit |

SECTION 4: THE GOLDEN RULE OF SUCCESS SEQUENCING

Your habits determine your behavior, but one thing is more important.

Focus.

Your attention is a form of currency that will either enrich or impoverish your life. That is why they call it 'paying attention.' Focus is the literal gateway to learning, reasoning, decision-making, problem-solving and perception.[28]

That is why consistent focus on your habits is the golden rule of success.

None of the people you have read about in this guide could have succeeded without an all-encompassing focus on their daily habits. Every individual here keeps a rigorous, personalized schedule that optimizes these habits.

Success, like your daily habits, is incredibly personal. Only you can

---

[28] Dr Taylor, Jim, Focus is The Gateway to Business Success, https://www.huffingtonpost.com/dr-jim-taylor/focus-is-the-gateway-to-b_b_4206552.html

decide when you have achieved a high enough level of success. And your habits are the stepping stones!

If you want to double your income, nothing is keeping you from it, but your habits. When you remove the bad and replace it with these powerful income-generating habits, you will immediately experience rapid change that will reshape your life.

That is why your primary focus must be a habitual practice, according to a personalized schedule. Without it, expect to fall back into bad patterns of behavior.

SECTION 5: THESE HABITS WILL MATTER MOST!

According to a study from Northwestern University, a domino effect happens when you adopt one lasting good habit.[29]

In other words, exercising every day will encourage positive eating habits. In turn, this may spread to you getting better quality sleep and performing better at work. Management of these small, seemingly insignificant habits starts with internalizing just one.

I want you to pick a habit from this list to act as your linchpin habit.

Then I want you to dedicate the next 66 days to internalizing that habit, and when you feel capable, adopt more from this list.

Even if you struggle to adopt more of these habits, I want you to commit to just the one. At no point over the next 66 days will you, at any point,

---

[29] Clear, James, How to Create a Chain Reaction of Good Habits, https://jamesclear.com/domino-effect

stop practicing that habit.

The first couple in this list have the most impact. They directly affect your daily performance. This is how you will naturally double your income in the short term.

Consider the domino effect active in you right now. But it is focused on negative habits. Switch to replacing them with positive habits, and you will soar!

The habits that matter most are the ones you learn to keep. Make them part of who you are, and soon you will leap an income bracket.

SECTION 6: WILLPOWER OR WONTPOWER: YOU DECIDE

The number 1 barrier to change is a mysterious thing called 'willpower.'

Those who have it are strong. Those who lack willpower are weak.

That is what we are taught to believe in our modern society. Your ability to resist short-term temptations is chalked up to your measure of willpower.

But you are never told what it is, or how to get it. How is it meant to take over, when you have no idea how it works?

Now I am going to lift the veil.

Willpower is little more than self-control. It is the conscious act of choosing what is right, over what is easy. It is picking cognition, over emotion. It is discipline.[30]

Willpower is a *habit*.

Right now, you habitually give in to your desires. What you need to do is replace this with your long-term plan for success. Say no to instant gratification!

Practice consciously choosing to focus on what is most important, every day.

If you don't want to exercise, use your willpower. Emotions drive your thoughts. Replace them with conscious thoughts that are more beneficial. You must exercise, to feel good today, tomorrow, this week. You must exercise to earn more and be better.

Practice willpower as a habit, and soon it will take over.

SECTION 7: REGAINING YOUR FAITH IN FREE WILL

'But I have so much to do.'

'I'll begin after my major project is over.'

'I'll just let this week pass, and I'll be ready.'

It is human nature to wait for the ideal time to change. You might have bought this guide with the intent to adopt these habits 'at some point.'

This is because you have lost faith in free will. Free will is your ability to choose between different courses of action, unimpeded. Now, life is all

---

[30] What You Need to Know About Willpower: The Psychological Science of Self-Control, http://www.apa.org/helpcenter/willpower.aspx

about impediments, but that does not mean you cannot choose to be better. You can.

We are all made up of a unique blend of strengths, weaknesses, circumstances and perceptions. Your free will must be exercised in accordance with your make-up, within your unique context, under your special circumstances.

The price of freedom is struggling.

The price of earning more is learning to be better.[31]

Then being better – every day!

If you cannot be better consistently, hope is lost.

In this way, free will gives you the opportunity to be whoever you want, as long as you are willing to go through the wringer to get there. It will be hard! If it were easy, everyone would be successful and living these rare lives.

My advice to be something is to practice.

Start and start *today*.

---

[31] Dr Schwartz, Seth, Do We Have Free Will,
https://www.psychologytoday.com/us/blog/proceed-your-own-risk/201311/do-we-have-free-will

Check Out Our Other AMAZING Titles:

1. Resolving Anxiety and Panic Attacks

A Guide to Overcoming Severe Anxiety, Controlling Panic Attacks and Reclaiming Your Life Again

Worldwide, one in six people is affected by a mental health disorder. So you are not alone in this (Ritchie & Roser, 2019). There is a difference between clinical anxiety and everyday anxiety. Everyday anxiety is normal and in often cases, it is necessary, while chronic anxiety will leave you functionally impaired. This book will not only inform you about anxiety and panic attacks but also introduce you to various methods and techniques that aid in getting rid of anxiety. It is a perfect package if you want to make long-lasting, meaningful changes in your life in a way that gets rid of anxiety. Knowledge is power, so gaining information about anxiety and panic attacks already puts you in the lead against them.

In the first chapter, we'll start with the basic knowledge of panic attacks and anxiety. The symptoms of both are pretty much the same, but there are some major differences as well. Knowing their difference and similarities can help you clearly understand your condition. Some basic ways of coping with them are also explained alongside their symptoms.

After gaining knowledge about anxiety and panic attacks in the first section, you will seek answers and ways to overcome them. The second chapter goes more in detail about the physical effects of anxiety. There are some types of anxiety which are also talked briefly about in the chapter. There are also therapies and treatments that are used to overcome and control anxiety. Their details are discussed in the chapter from where you can figure out what sort of treatment will suit you better. Some other ways of coping with anxiety are also discussed and they will surely prove beneficial to the reader.

The third chapter will make you aware of how interrelated physical and mental healths are. There are also details on how to improve one's physical health to influence a person's anxiety positively. You will also learn how important practicing well-being is. If you are to ignore physical health, it will cause problems for your mental health as well.

The fourth chapter will delve deep into mindfulness and its vast benefits. Mindfulness is a very powerful tool we have but don't know how to use. It can be practiced through meditation techniques, etc. It makes us see things more clearly than ever before. Practicing Mindfulness will arm you against any anxiety and panic attacks. In this chapter, it is explained in detail what it means and what are its advantages.

In the fifth chapter, we will learn about meditation and how can it help manage anxiety. We first start off by knowing what it is. You also have got to know its benefits and various techniques from which one can pick according to their choice. We will also learn the accurate posture you should have during meditation. We will learn how mediation reinforces our brain to stave off anxiety and panic attacks. It is a long road but a successful one for sure. Besides helping us out with anxiety and panic disorder, meditation has numerous other benefits for our body and mind.

The sixth chapter will explore the meaning behind self-love and its importance in fighting anxiety. Our battle with anxiety has to start from a positive ground. We first have to be fully comfortable and respectful towards ourselves. You will also find out how lack of self-love can actually breed anxiety.

Opening about anxiety is not an easy task but could be very helpful against anxiety. How to go about the whole process is talked about in detail in the seventh chapter. You will also learn how to evaluate your therapist and choose the right one. In this chapter, there are also guidelines for people who have just recently become aware of their anxiety and now they want to seek help. It will give them knowledge about things to consider when talking to someone about mental health, what you should accept and be prepared for. There is also information about talk therapy there.

In the eighth chapter, we address the misunderstanding about anxiety. Despite affecting so many people, it remains a different experience for all of them. There are also common mistakes pointed out in that chapter which we'll go into detail the mistakes that make our anxiety worse.

The ninth chapter is about where we talk about putting our foot down and start to incorporate practices into our life which will help you get rid of anxiety and panic attacks. We will learn how to manage our responses. It is basically a comprehensive listing of all the things you should be avoiding or adapting to lead a healthy lifestyle free of anxiety.

*Want to read more? Purchase our book on **Anxiety and Panic Attacks** today!*

2. Cognitive Behavioral Therapy

How CBT Can Be Used to Rewire Your Brain, Stop Anxiety, and Overcome Depression

Cognitive stems from cognition, which encapsulates the idea of how we learn and the knowledge that we carry. The things you learn are part of your cognition, and what you do with that information is included in that category as well. Cognition includes a wide list of information that you might not fully realize.

Behavior is what we do. It is how we act. The things that you choose to say to other people are all about your behavior. How you react to what others have to say will exhibit your behavior as well. Your behavior is all about your mind interacting with your body and how that interacts with the people and other things that surround you.

Therapy is any form of help, usually from a trained professional, to help improve on whatever the therapy is specified for. You might get physical therapy to help regain strength in your knee after having a serious surgery. You can also get therapy to help overcome an alcohol or drug addiction.

Throughout this book, we're going to give you the basis you need to start understanding cognitive behavioral therapy. The three together—cognitive, behavioral, therapy—all make up CBT, which is a method that is going to directly help you overcome the mental illness that you are hoping to treat.

Therapy can be expensive, and even if you do have the means to go through with this process, you might struggle to find the right therapist. Sometimes, you might live in an area where there is only one therapist within a close distance, but you don't have a vibe with them that you find to be helpful. You might also find that you are desperate for help and that you want a therapist, but insurance coverage isn't always good for this.

By reading this book, you'll be able to find the tools you need to help with overcoming your most challenging thoughts. We are going to take you through the steps to identify the root issues and come up with specific methods to get you through.

Want to read more? Purchase our book on **Cognitive Behavioral Therapy** *today!*

3. Effective Guide On How to Sleep Well Everyday

The Easy Method For Better Sleep, Insomnia And Chronic Sleep Problems

"A well spent day brings happy sleep." — *Leonardo da Vinci*

Are you experiencing the worst restless feeling? Has your doctor diagnosed you with insomnia, restlessness, sleeplessness? When the whole world around you seems to be in peaceful deep slumber, you are the one who is restless. No matter what term is used to describe it, the fact is that it is you who is actually going through insomnia, and nothing could feel worse than that.

So you drag yourself from bed in the morning feeling as earth, with its entire lock stock and barrel, has decided to perch on your head for the day. Yet you go through the motions of the day, though you barely manage to make it through the hours. By the early night, you fall on to bed hoping this night will be different because you're dead tired and nothing will keep you from sleeping like a log. It's 2.00 a.m. now, dawn is breaking through and there you are, still wide awake and ready to scream to the world because no matter how tired you are or how hard you have tried, you simply can't get to sleep.

While there are proven facts and evidence of the devastating effects of sleeping less, the investigations are still on to establish the exact nature of effects resulting from too much sleep. Some researchers argue that people who sleep much longer than necessarily have a higher death rate. Physical and mental conditions such as depression or socioeconomic status can also lead to excessive sleep. There are other researchers who argue that the human body will naturally restrain it from sleeping more hours than really necessary. However, with research still underway for concrete evidence of the effects of over sleeping the best path you can choose is to adopt a sleeping pattern somewhere in the middle. According to the National Sleep Foundation, this middle range falls between seven and eight hours of sleep during the night. Despite these statistics, the best way to ensure you receive sufficient sleeping time is to let your own body act as your guide. You can always sleep a little extra if you feel exhausted or sleep a little less than usual if you feel you are oversleeping.

Dangers of Sleep deprivation.

Though sleep is something the average human being takes for granted, it is also one of the greatest mysteries in life. Just like we still don't have all the answers to the quantum field or gravity, researchers are still exploring the reasons behind the 'whats' and 'whys' of sleep. However, one fact unchallenged about sleep is that a proper sleep is paramount for maintaining good health. The general guideline regarding the optimal amount of sleep for an adult range from six to eight hours! If you carry on with too little or too much of this general guideline you are exposing yourself to the risk of adverse health effects.

Though sleep is something that comes naturally to many people, the problems of sleep deprivation have today become a pressing problem with more and more people succumbing to chronic sleeping disorders. Unfortunately, a great number of these people do not even realize that lack of sleep or sleep deprivation is at the root of their manifold problems in life. Scientific research also points out that lack of sleep on a continuous scale can lead to severe repercussions on your health.

If you have been experiencing impaired sleep patterns for a longer period, you also face the risk of:

- Severely impairing your immunity strength

- Promoting the risk of tumor growth, as it has been scientifically established that a tumor can grow at least two to three times faster among animals subjected to severe sleeping dysfunctions within a laboratory setting.

- Creating a pre-diabetic condition in the body. Insomnia creates hunger, making you want to eat even when you have already had a meal. This situation can lead to problems of obesity in turn.

- Critically impairing memory. How many times during the day have you found it difficult to remember even the most mundane and repetitive events when you have had no more than 4 – 5 hours of sleep? Even a single night of impaired sleep plays havoc with our memory faculties, just think what it can do to your brain if you consistently lose sleep.

- Ruining your performance level both physically and mentally as your problem-solving abilities will not be working in peak order.

- Stomach ulcers

- Constipation, hemorrhoids

- Heart diseases

- Depression, lethargy and other mood disorders

- Daytime drowsiness

- Irritability

- Low energy

- Low mental clarity

- Reaction time slows down

- Lower productivity

- More accidents and mistakes

- Lower levels of growth hormone and testosterone

The growth hormone in the body which is vital for maintaining our looks, energy, and skin texture is produced by the pituitary gland. The specialty of this hormone production procedure is that it is only produced during the times of deep slumber or during intense workout sessions. In the absence of normal production of the growth hormone, our bodies will start on a premature aging process. According to research, people suffering from chronic insomnia are three times more susceptible to contract fatal diseases. When you lose sleep overnight, you cannot make up for it by sleeping more the next day. A night's lost sleep will be lost forever. More alarmingly if you continue to lose sleep regularly, they will create a cumulative negative effect that will disrupt your general health. All in all, sleeping deficiencies can effectively make your life miserable, as you already know.

How Much Sleep Do I Really Need?

This is a question that remains a mystery just like the questions of why and what makes us want to sleep. In response to a question of how many hours of sleep do we really need, an expert has answered that it is actually lot less than what we have been taught. On the other hand, though a good night's sleep is vital for good health, overdoing the sleeping can be equally bad for us. But if you sleep less and continue this for too long, the result will be confusion between body and brain signals, resulting in muddled thoughts, lethargic feelings, and overall lassitude. So, the question remains, how many hours of sleep do we really need? Is it essential to sleep the prescribed number of eight hours a day or is catching up a good sleep on a five to six-hour basis enough?

The eight hours of sleep theory is increasingly becoming unpractical in this fast-paced lifestyle. Actually, the recommendation of eight hours of sleep arises based on the idea that our ancestors had their beauty sleep between 8-9 hours in the past. In today's context, this concept is regarded more or less as a myth. In a study conducted by the Sleep Research Center, youngsters within the age group of 8 to 17 generally sleep for about nine hours during the night. However, in the case of adults, this theory is not applicable as a majority of them are sleepless and many of them thrive after a solid sleep varying between 5-7 hours.

A research conducted by the National Institute of Health has established that people who sleep soundly for nine hours a day or more are actually two times more vulnerable than those who sleep less in developing

Parkinson's disease. A study report released by the Diabetes Care states that people claiming to sleep less than five hours or more than nine hours daily are the ones with the highest risk of attracting diabetes. In contrast, a large number of contemporary studies prove that people with sleeping patterns that do not exceed or fall beyond seven hours daily possess the highest survival rate. The persons who experience sleeping disorders and sleep less than 4.5 hours have the worst survival rate.

When ascertaining the correct number of hours you should sleep, the fact is that there is no magic number of hours. It will depend on a person to person basis as well as factors like age, activity, and performance level. For example, smaller children and teenagers require more sleep compared to adults. Your personal requirements will not be the same as your friend or colleague who is of the same age and gender as you. Because your sleep needs are unique and individual. According to the National Sleep Foundation, the difference of sleep requirements between two people of the same age, gender, and activity level is due to their basal sleep needs and sleep debt.

Your basal sleep need is the number of hours of sleep you typically need to engage in optimal performance levels. The sleep debt comprises of the accumulated number of hours of sleep you have lost as a result of poor sleeping habits, a recent sickness, social demands, environmental factors, etc. A healthy adult generally possesses a basal sleep need between seven and eight hours each night. If you have experienced sleeping difficulties and as a result accumulated a sleep debt you will find that your performance level is not up to its usual standard, even if you wake up after seven or eight hours of restful sleep. The symptoms will be most apparent during the times the circadian rhythm naturally alters like during mid-afternoon or overnight. One of the ways of easing out of an accumulated sleep debt situation is to get a few extra hours of sleep for a couple of nights until you regain your natural sleeping rhythm and vitality during the day.

Understand what Kind of a Sleeper Are You?

Sleep, dear reader, is the precious restorative that rights so many physical and mental wrongs. The elixir that transforms life and puts a spring in your step, a smile on your face, and the feeling that you can take care of everything that comes your way is sleep. Undervalued, ignored, and forgotten until you wake up to the realization that it's one of the essential foundations of daily wellbeing.

So what kind of a sleeper are you? There are many studies and descriptions of how we sleep but the common consensus settles for the following five simple categories:

1. Lively, healthy early risers!

These happy individuals usually get the sleep they need and rarely feel exhausted or fatigued. They are typically younger than the other groups, usually married or with a long-term partner, working full-time and definitely a morning person with no serious medical conditions.

2. Relaxed and retired seniors.

This is the oldest group in the survey with half of the sample being 65 or older. They sleep the most with an average of 7.3 hours per night compared to 6.8 across all groups. Sleep disorders are rare even though there is a significant proportion with at least one medical disorder.

3. Dozing drones.

These busy people are usually married/partnered and employed but they often work much longer than forty hours a week. Frequently working up to the hour when they go to bed, they get up early so they're always short of sleep and struggle to keep up with the daily pressures of life. Statistically, they'll feel tired or fatigued at least three days a week.

4. Galley slaves.

This group works the longest hours and often suffers from weight problems as well as an unhealthy reliance on caffeine to get through the day. Shift workers often fall into this group and there is also a marked tendency to be a night owl or evening person. They get the least amount of sleep and are more likely to take naps yet, surprisingly, this group often believes that, despite the state of their health, they are getting enough sleep.

5. Insomniacs.

Here is the largest proportion of night people and many of them quite rightly believe they have a sleep problem. About half of this group feel they get less sleep than they need and the same proportion admits to feeling tired, fatigued and lacking energy most of the time.

So, which of the five groups do you think you fit into?

If you're a happy member of Group One, your sleep should by definition be absolutely fine. Don't worry. We've got some really good ideas to share with you to keep you right on track and we'll even add some special extra features to your nightly rest routine to maximize the experience. If you're not in this group, our aim is to help you become a full-time member of the healthy, happy sleepers' association! Membership is for life.

Group Three represents too many tired, irritable, and generally inefficient individuals whose quality of life is impaired because they're too tired too often. Their work suffers because they rarely have sufficient rest to successfully assimilate the day's events. Their home life is degraded because work intrudes too often and they're just too tired to enjoy the pleasures and comfort of a life away from work. Feeling tired becomes their default position and they know they need to do something to give their minds and bodies the rest they deserve. Individuals in this group frequently suffer from long- term mental, physical and emotional stress.

The fourth group is rightly described as the night owls. They work the longest hours and, as we noted above, they typically work shifts. The health problems associated with this group include a marked tendency towards obesity as well as a range of inflammatory diseases. Despite the fact that these people rarely look or feel well, they seem to ignore the evidence and usually claim to get enough sleep, relying on sugary energy drinks and caffeine to keep them awake during waking hours. They take naps because their bodies can't function without additional sleep during the day. An objective analysis of their health would typically reveal a range of health and wellbeing issues.

Insomniacs are the dominant members of Group Five, people who don't get enough sleep, can't get to sleep, and who know they have a problem. Unfortunately, many insomniacs end up taking prescription medication to deal with their symptoms and we have to question the benefits of this solution in light of the many unpleasant side effects associated with long-term sleeping pill dependency. For insomniacs, life is a constant struggle because of the accumulative effects of long-term sleep deprivation.

Health issues abound, depression becomes a major risk, their ability to function normally is often impaired, and they lose sight of their potential to deal successfully with life's daily challenges. They sometimes refer to their condition as living in a nightmare world where they are constantly exhausted and simply cannot function. It's completely understandable that a doctor would prescribe sleeping drugs because the dangers of sleep deprivation can be acute.

Before we begin to examine the practicalities of sleep, we need to know how much sleep is appropriate for each of us as individuals. It's not surprising that different age groups have different sleep requirements.

For example, very young children and infants can sleep in total for around 14 - 15 hours a day. And if you've got teenagers, you might have guessed that adolescents usually need more sleep than adults. Teens can easily sleep between 8.5 to 9.5 hours a night.

It's widely understood that during the first trimester, pregnant women often find they need a lot more sleep than usual. The fact is that if you feel tired during the day, find yourself yawning or taking a nap, you're short on sleep. And this is the time for you to do something practical, realistic, and effective to take care of the problem.

There are many myths surrounding the condition known as OAS or Obstructive Sleep Apnea. It's estimated that around 18 million Americans suffer from the condition but the numbers could be much higher because many people don't report the condition to their doctors. This condition is far more than just loud snoring, although snoring can be a sign of sleep apnea.

People with this condition skip breathing 400 times during the night. The delay in breathing can last from ten to thirty seconds and is then followed by a loud snore as breathing suddenly resumes. The normal sleep cycle is interrupted and this can leave sufferers feeling tired and exhausted during the day. It is a serious condition, especially since it can lead to accidents at work, problems when driving, as well as increasing the risk of heart attacks and strokes. It can affect people of all ages, including children, but tends to affect people more after the age of forty.

Weight also plays a part and there is evidence that shedding excess pounds can improve the condition. Despite all the advice and overwhelming evidence, there are still surprising numbers of sleep apnea sufferers who continue to smoke. Smoking is a perfect way to increase the severity and risks of this debilitating condition.

If you've already trimmed your weight, quit smoking and tried sleeping on your side but still suffer from the condition, you need to see your doctor. There are many treatments available including a special mask that delivers constant air flow to keep the breathing passage open. Lifestyle choices can clearly make a positive difference, too.

Your body, your brain, your mind and your emotional functioning all rely on sufficient sleep to operate efficiently. If you don't get enough sleep, everything suffers. Research suggests that it's much harder than you might imagine to adapt having less sleep than your body needs. The sleep deficit has to be repaid at some point or we'll experience increasingly severe problems.

Simple techniques of preparing for bed

1. Try to get to bed early. The recharging of the body's adrenal system usually takes place between 11p.m. and 1a.m. in the morning. The gallbladder uses the same time to release the toxin build up in the body. If you happen to be awake when both these functions are taking place within your body, there is the possibility of the toxin backing up to the liver which can endanger your health very badly. Sleeping late are byproducts of

modern living styles. However, the human body was created in synchronization of nature and its activities. That is why before the advent of electricity people used to go to bed just after sundown and wake up with sunrise.

2. Don't alter your bedtimes haphazardly. Try to stick to a pattern where you go to bed and wake up at the same time. This should be done even on weekends. The continuous pattern will help your body to fit into a rhythm.

3. Maintain a soothing bedtime routine. This can change from person to person. You can use deep breathing exercises, meditation, use of aromatherapy, a gentle relaxing massage given by your partner, or even going through a complete and relaxing skin care routine. The secret is to get into a rhythm which makes you comfortable, relaxed, and ready for bed. Repeating it every day will help in easing out the tensions of the day.

4. Refrain from taking any heavy fluids two hours before bed time. This habit will minimize the number of times you need to visit the bathroom in the middle of the night. You should also make a habit of going to the bathroom just before you get into bed, so that you will not get the urge during night time.

5. Eat a meal enriched with proteins several hours before your bed time. The protein will enhance the production of L-tryptophan which is essential for the production of serotonin and melatonin. Follow up your meal with some fruit to help the tryptophan to cross easily across the blood brain barrier.

6. Refrain from taking any snacks while in bed or just before bed and reduce the level of sugar and grains in your dinner time as it

will raise the blood sugar level, delaying sleep. When the body starts metabolizing these elements and the blood sugar level start dropping you will find yourself suddenly awake and unable to go back to sleep.

7. A hot bath before bed is found to be very soothing. When the body temperature is stimulated to a raised level during late evening by the time you get into bed, it will be ready to drop, signaling slumber time to your brain.

8. Stop your work and put them away ideally one to two hours before bed. The interval between work and bedtime should be used for unwinding from the pressure and tension of work. It is essential that you approach your bed with a calm mind instead of being hyped up about some matter.

9. If you prefer reading, a novel with an uplifting story instead of a stimulating one like suspense or mystery is recommended. Or the suspense will keep you up half the night awake trying to visualize the end to the mystery!

A Few Lifestyle Suggestions to Make You Sleep Better

Don't take medications and drugs unless it is absolutely necessary for your health and wellbeing. A majority of prescribed and over the counter drugs can cause changes in your sleeping patterns.

Avoid drinks with alcohol or caffeine. Caffeine takes longer to metabolize in the body so that your body will experience its effects much longer after consumption. That is why even the cup of coffee you had in the evening will keep you awake during the night. Some of the medications and drugs in the market also contain caffeine which account for their capacity to generate sleeping irregularities. Though alcohol can make you feel drowsy the effect is very much short lived. Once the feeling goes away, you will find that sleep is eluding you for many hours and even the sleep that you finally reach will not take you to deep slumber after alcohol. In the absence of deep sleep, your body will not be able to perform its usual healing and regeneration process is vital for lasting healthiness.

Engage in regular exercise activities. If you are contained in an 8-hour office job, you should make sure that your body receives plenty of exercise which can dramatically increase your sleep health. The best time to exercise is, however, not closer to your bedtime but in the morning.

Keep away from sensitive food types that will keep you awake at night like sugar, pasteurized dairy foods, and grains. These foods can result in congestion, leading to gastric disorders.

The sleep apnea risk is enhanced amongst people with weight issues. If you think you have gained a few extra pounds and during this time you have also experienced sleeping trouble focus on losing the extra weight as a priority. The sleeping issue will correct automatically.

If your body is going through a hormone upheaval like during menopausal or premenopausal time, seek advice from your family physician, as this time can lead to sleeping difficulties.

Want to read more? Purchase our book on **Effective Guide On How to Sleep Well Everyday** *today!*

Made in the USA
Middletown, DE
30 July 2021

45056555R00080